THE

REAL

SECRETS

OF

BEAUTY

INTERNATIONAL IMAGE PRESS

THE

REAL

SECRETS

OF

BEAUTY

Diane H. Irons

Publisher: International Image Press

Library of Congress Catalog Card Number: 93-91790

ISBN 0-9639394-0-8

Cover Design by Kimberlee Florez

Manufactured in the United States of America

This book is dedicated to my beloved sons
Keith and Kirk
for teaching me the Secret of Real Beauty

CONTENTS

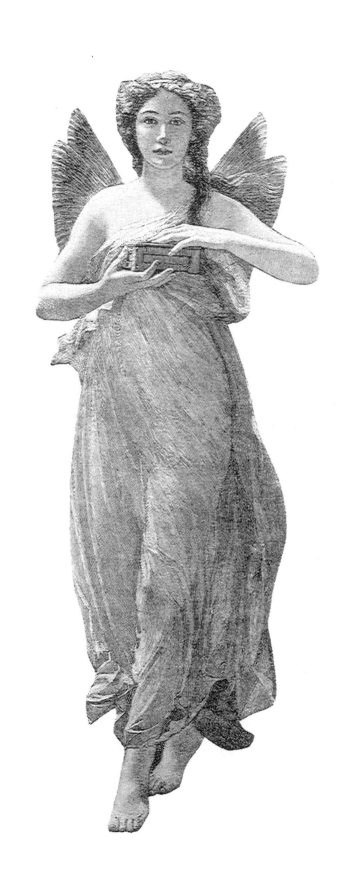

INTRODUCTION

From my work as a Radio/TV and Print
journalist, I have constantly taken a consumer
oriented view towards the subject of beauty
itself. My work has been in both spectrums.
From my years as a model/agent, I have tried to
approach beauty with a discerning and
objective eye.

What I have discovered across the board is that
"Real" beauty is not expensive, nor is it
elusive. It is the result of self respect
and self acceptance.

Real beauty is an ancient art, and very much
part of our feminine nature. The bashing
of beauty has come from rituals gone awry.

In its proper perspective, being the best
you can be physically, is as important
as being the best you can be emotionally,
intellectually, and spiritually.

It is my hope that this book will teach
you to take charge of your looks. It is never
too late, and it is certainly never to
early to enjoy your true feminine nature.
Beauty is our birthright.

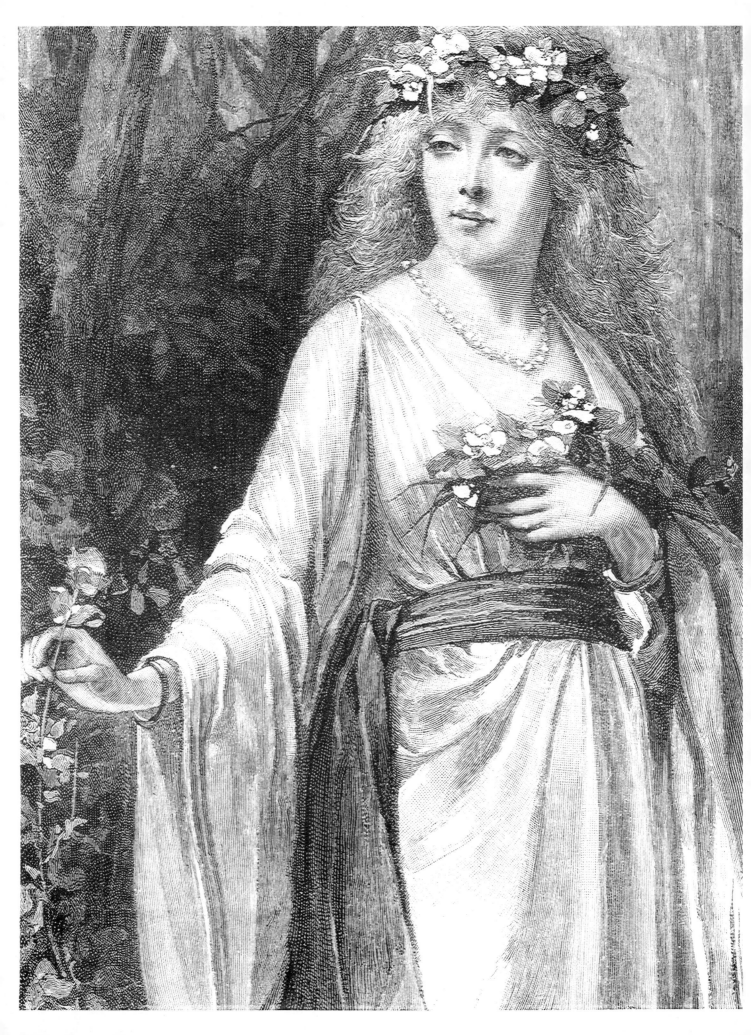

CHAPTER ONE

SECRETS OF

ATTITUDE

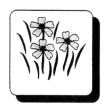

Almost everything we do is done on appearance.
The pursuit of beauty is as old as time.
Cute babies are held longer.
We love flowers for their "beauty".

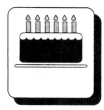

**THE LESS YOU THINK ABOUT AGING,
THE YOUNGER YOU WILL STAY.
STAY YOUNG AT HEART FOREVER!**

*Beauty begins with self acceptance.
Look in the mirror and just say
HI!*

Take pride in yourself. You don't have to be a
fashion plate every waking moment, but give yourself
the self respect you deserve.

Don't get stuck in time.
Keep reinventing yourself.
Keep changing.

Each day, do something that is just for you.
* Give yourself a spa treatment
* Buy a favorite food to nourish your body
* Enjoy that special tea

LEARN TO VALUE YOURSELF

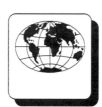

Know when to let go.   You're not in charge of the universe.

Keep a scrapbook of goals.
Start a journal.

RETURN TO ELEGANCE. IT TAKES JUST A FEW
SECONDS TO LIGHT CANDLES FOR DINNER.
MANY GREAT BEAUTIES, ESPECIALLY EUROPEANS,
ENJOY A GLASS OF WINE BEFORE DINNER.
NOT ONLY IS IT CONSIDERED CIVILIZED, BUT IS
REPORTED TO REDUCE THE RISK OF HEART DISEASE.

Some beauties report that enjoying one glass of wine before dinner relaxes
them to the extent that they actually eat less during mealtime.

Know when it's time to make a change.
> *Hair style*
> *Makeup*
> *Even your surroundings*

LESS IS MORE!
> **In makeup, hair, dress, etc.**
> **You can make your mark quietly and elegantly.**

Show your originality!
Try to remember what compliments
have been repeated about you through
the years .

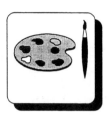

PLAY UP THOSE FEATURES!

****

AVOID NEGATIVES IN LIFE WHEN YOU CAN.
THIS INCLUDES PEOPLE, PLACES, AND THINGS
THAT DEPLETE YOUR ENERGY AND CAUSE
YOU ANXIETY.

****

CHOOSE A BEAUTY MENTOR.
Learn ALL her tricks.

Visualize your goal. See yourself as:
        Slimmer
        Younger
        More assertive
        Happier

****

Try to stay in line with your own unique energy level.
Take breaks.   Eat every four hours.

****

BEAUTY BEGINS WITH SELF ACCEPTANCE.
Love yourself and your loved ones will benefit.

****

Try to find HUMOR in every aspect of your life.

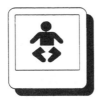

EVERY CHILD BELIEVES SHE IS THE CENTER OF
THE UNIVERSE UNLESS TOLD OTHERWISE

Children live what they are told.
It goes with them throughout their lives.
If there is a word that has been with you:

FAT

UGLY

LAZY

Now is the time to take that word
and throw it away!

YOUR REFUSAL TO OWN THAT WORD
IS YOUR FIRST STEP BACK TO THE TRUE
BEAUTY THAT IS YOUR BIRTHRIGHT.

SELF PORTRAIT

Drawings are our subconscious speaking to us.
Take a pencil or crayon and draw a picture of yourself.
Look at it.

Ask yourself what your drawing says about you.

1. DID YOU TAKE UP THE WHOLE PAGE?
2. ARE YOU IN THE CORNER?
3. ARE ANY OF YOUR BODY PARTS MISSING?
4. ARE YOU WEARING CLOTHES?
5. WHAT KIND OF CLOTHES ARE YOU WEARING?
6. ARE YOU WEARING SHOES?
7. ARE ANY OF YOUR BODY PARTS OUT OF PROPORTION?
8. WHAT WOULD YOU NAME YOUR DRAWING?

When I speak to groups or work with clients, I use this test. It tells me
what I need to know in order to help them with their image/esteem issues. More
importantly, the questions are phrased so that the answers are self-evident.

THE MOST REVEALING SELF PORTRAIT RESULTS?

TEENS & HOMEMAKERS RE-ENTERING THE WORKPLACE

THEY WERE THE MOST LIKELY TO DRAW THEMSELVES WITHOUT
BODY PARTS, GROTESQUE BODY PARTS, OR OCCUPYING A SMALL
CORNER OF THE PAGE.

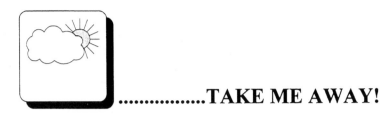 ....**TAKE ME AWAY!**

Here's a handy way to use up that suntan oil in your closet.

AFTER A BATH OR SHOWER, REPLACE YOUR
USUAL OIL WITH YOUR FAVORITE SUNTAN LOTION.
NOT ONLY WILL IT MOISTURIZE YOUR SKIN,
BUT IT WILL REMIND YOU OF THOSE BALMY
CAREFREE BEACH DAYS.

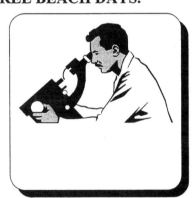

BEAUTY IS A SCIENCE OF THE MIND.

Replace the words younger, thinner, firmer, smarter, etc. with:

<u>BETTER</u>

Have someone videotape you. It will give you information about posture, weight, hair, demeanor, and other insights that a mirror or photo cannot reveal.

WHAT YOU WEAR IS LESS IMPORTANT THAN *HOW* YOU WEAR IT.

Dare to do something different whether it's getting a pedicure, manicure, or highlighting your hair.   Of course, you can always change back.

ALWAYS ACCEPT COMPLIMENTS GRACEFULLY AND THEN WRITE THEM DOWN!

Establish standards for yourself.

DEVELOP YOUR OWN UNIQUE STYLE, BUT KEEP UP TO DATE BY PURCHASING ONE TRENDY ITEM A SEASON.

The body is as great a miracle as the mind.

Sometimes beauty is not in the eye, but in the heart of the admirer.

NEVER KEEP OR WEAR ANYTHING YOU DON'T LIKE.

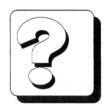

Does beauty matter?
69% of what will remain in people's minds about you will
happen in the first 8 to 10 seconds of non verbal contact

FORGIVE YOURSELF

When you break your diet   When you overspend
When you waste a day

THEN GET ON WITH YOUR LIFE

DON'T THINK OF YOUR BEAUTY RITUALS AS OPPRESSIVE,
BUT AS A FORM OF MEDITATION.

BE YOUR OWN TEACHER
Close your eyes and go back to that time
        *When you first felt really good about your body
        * When you first felt badly about your looks

SECRETS

"I maintain my looks by maintaining my posture.   It
doesn't matter what I am wearing, it looks better when
my back is straight and my tummy is tucked in."

JAN, 28/MODEL

"Keeping only one area in my home that is dedicated
to my beauty regimens keeps me more organized as well
more time efficient."

ANGELA, 41/ARTIST

"The first thing that I do after undressing is to wipe off
my shoes and mend, air out, and get my outfit ready for
the next wearing. It saves me time and aggravation
every time!"

DONNA, 45/STEWARDESS

"Polish and protect every purchase and save lots of money
in the long run."

BRENDA, 51/SALES

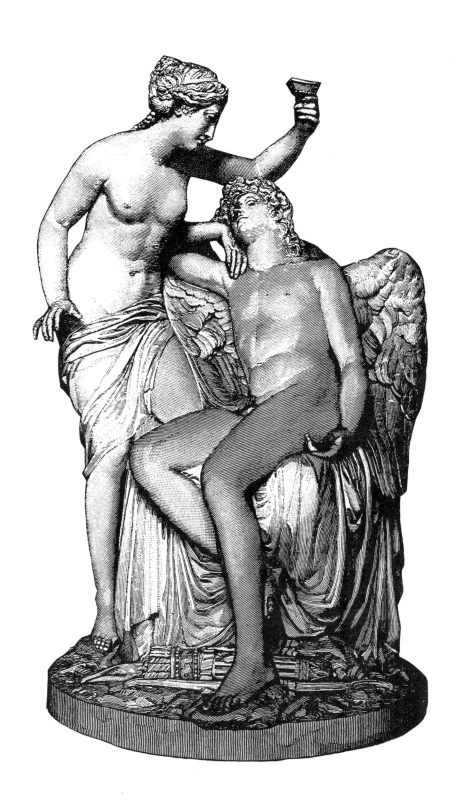

CHAPTER

TWO

SECRETS

OF

HISTORY'S

BEAUTIES

DUPLICATE CLEOPATRA'S BATHING RITUAL.
Use one cup powdered dry milk under running bath water
and soak away your dry skin.

*CATHERINE DE MEDICI REPORTEDLY HAD ALMOST 200 MIRRORS
IN HER CHATEAUS*
Of course, you won't collect that many, but mirrors are a great
source of light and allow you to keep track of your own looks.

**MARIE ANTOINETTE GAVE AWAY HER BEAUTY SECRET FOR
BEAUTIFUL SKIN JUST BEFORE SHE WENT TO THE GUILLOTINE**
PS: She told her lady-in-waiting it was camphor oil and
water.   She used it on her face to keep her spectacular
skin moist and smooth.

IN THE ELIZABETHAN ERA, LADIES OF THE COURT WORE RED PAINT ON THEIR EYES.

UNTIL THE EARLY 1900'S COSMETICS WERE LACED WITH ARSENIC.

**Women in the 1800's developed severe stomach ailments
from wearing tightly laced corsets.**

SARAH BERNHARDT WAS A FRENCH BEAUTY AND FAMOUS ACTRESS WHO LIVED IN THE EARLY TWENTIETH CENTURY.

Her flamboyant style shocked the puritanical Victorians.

* Wore vivid colors
* Flaunted an eccentric lifestyle
* Made the use of heavy cosmetics fashionable again
* Used butter to keep her hands soft

ELIZABETH I, QUEEN OF ENGLAND

* Shaved her forehead to emphasis her hairline
* Painted her veins to accentuate her paleness
* Applied a form of lard to her red hair

IN THE 1920'S FASHIONABLE FLAPPERS CHEWED A SPECIAL FORMULA GUM TO LOSE WEIGHT.

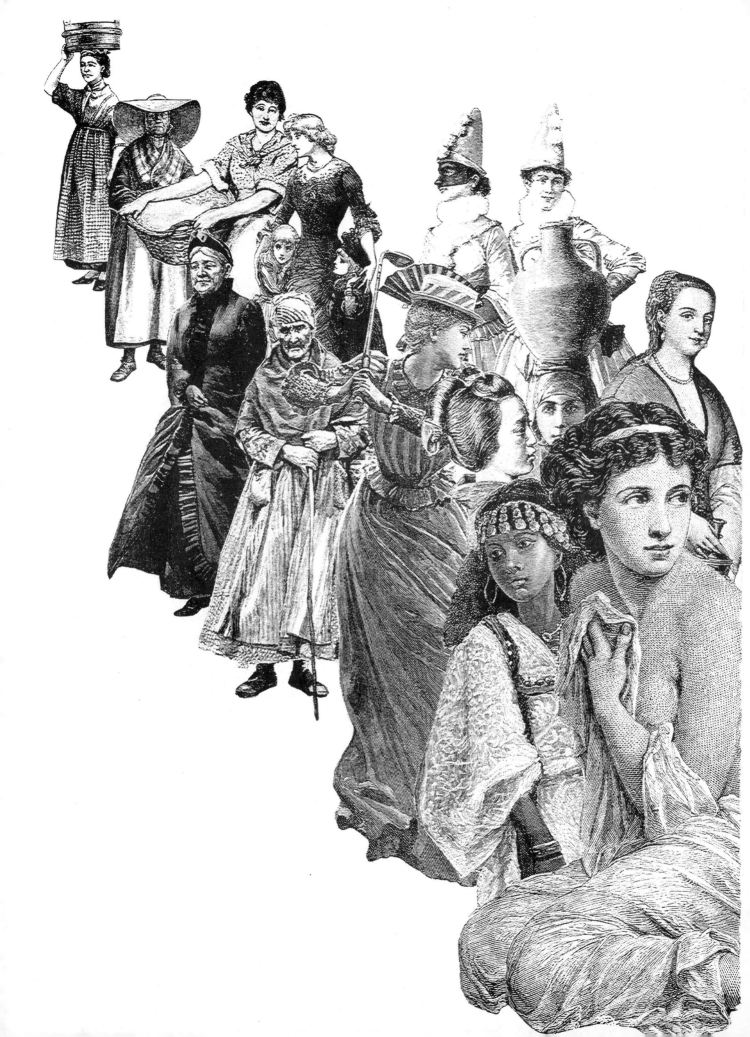

CHAPTER

THREE

SECRETS OF

INTERNATIONAL

BEAUTY

BLACK IS THE BASIS OF EVERY FRENCH WOMAN'S WARDROBE.

****

*   IN EUROPE FACE LIFTS ARE DONE MORE MODERATELY TO ACHIEVE A MORE NATURAL LOOK.

*   MORE BREAST REDUCTIONS ARE PERFORMED IN FRANCE THAN AUGMENTATIONS.

****

European men think women are absolutely perfect at the age of forty.

****

SCARVES AND SHAWLS ARE EVERYDAY ACCESSORIES THROUGHOUT WESTERN EUROPE

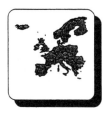

Not only do European women wear more jewelry, but they wear it more imaginatively.

JAPANESE WOMEN

- are quicker to adopt trends than Americans
- love body hugging fashions
- adore hats
- consider beauty part of wellness
- wear whitening cream under their foundation
- use facial blotting papers to remove oil

Europeans place more importance on skin care than on cosmetics, and spend more money on skin care products than on their makeup.

FRENCH WOMEN SELDOM USE SOAP, PREFERRING TO WASH WITH FACIAL CLEANSERS INSTEAD.

THE ELEGANT EUROPEAN STILL TANS HER FACE FAR TOO MUCH!

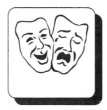

Most European women think that American women apply their makeup in such a heavy manner that it looks "like a mask".

SECRETS

The following advice comes from American models working in Paris.

"Take a white tee shirt and wear it under everything from
   suits to jeans."

"Use a couple of brooches to nip in an oversized jacket."

"I have learned to take an old cardigan and dress it up
   with lace, jewelry, you name it, and wear it under
   absolutely everything!   At night I wear it backwards."

"It seems that I am not completely dressed until I adorn a
   scarf.   I wear one in my hair, tie it on my purse, and
   even wrap more than one around my waist."

"I spent a lot of money on a trench coat, but I find that
   it takes me everywhere.   I layer it according to
   the weather situation. It's big and chic and was well
   worth the extra money."

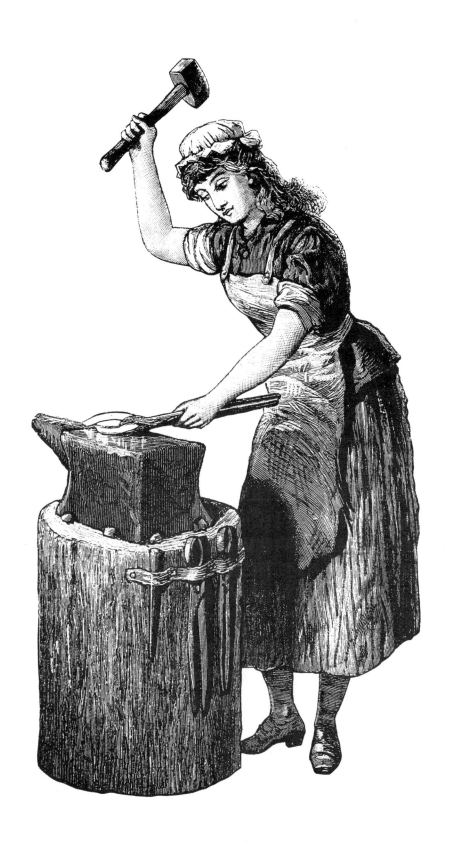

CHAPTER FOUR

SECRETS OF

MAINTENANCE

You take care of your car and your home. Why wouldn't you give yourself that same consideration? It takes only minutes a day and will add so much to your self esteem. The women who seem so absolutely and perfectly put together do not spend as much time as we think on their beauty regimes.
What they have learned to do is to streamline their routines by staying with what works, and choosing products that are multi purpose.

FOR INSTANCE: When you brush your teeth, brush your jewelry. Forget expensive sonic cleaners and messy jewelry dips. Even Joan Rivers cleans her jewelry with toothpaste.

Don't forget to brush your TONGUE (for good hygiene), and your LIPS (to exfoliate) when you get that toothbrush out!

Great beauties have the self confidence to use what works FOR THEM. They don't need the ego reinforcement of paying over-inflated department store prices.

REAL LIFE BEAUTIES ESTABLISH ROUTINES THAT
THEY USE THROUGHOUT THEIR LIVES. DOING SOMETHING
OVER AND OVER AGAIN MAKES IT:

1. <u>EASY</u>
   If you know that you are going to cleanse, tone,
   and moisturize every single morning, you do
   it without even thinking about it.

2. <u>HABIT</u>
   The beauties I interviewed stated that there is
   an almost addictive quality to their regimes.
   A feeling that the day was not complete if
   something was left out was most often mentioned.

Although I mentioned that the women I interviewed were confident in using
products that worked for them regardless of price, they also stated that
they were not afraid to spend extra money on certain services and goods.
Here's a rundown on what they did and why:

1. HAIR
   Real beauties never seem to have a "bad hair day"
   This is because they rarely go beyond 6 to 8 weeks
   between cuts. This applied to hair that is long or short.

HAIR SHOULD BE THE LEAST OF YOUR BEAUTY CONCERNS.
THE MOST YOU SHOULD HAVE TO DO, NO MATTER WHAT
LENGTH IS MOST COMFORTABLE, IS TOWEL DRY, BLOW DRY
AND COMB THROUGH.   GEL OR MOUSSE SEEMS TO BE THE
STYLING TOOL OF CHOICE.

2. FOUNDATION

The same beauties stating their confidence in using lesser priced products claimed that one area in which they would not skimp was foundation. Foundations most mentioned were *Alexandra De Markoff* and *Chanel.*

HIGHER PRICED FOUNDATIONS SEEM TO GIVE MORE BANG FOR YOUR BUCK. THE ONES I TESTED WENT ON MORE SMOOTHLY AND PROVIDED BETTER COVERAGE.

3. CLOTHING BASICS

For basic pieces like a black skirt, career suit, handbag, and shoes, Real Beauties invested in designer or couture lines. These pieces were interspersed with lower lines, the so called *TRENDY* items.

4. COLORS

Basic colors were mentioned as the ones that women were accustomed to paying more. This was the case with major accessories and clothing purchases (black was the color most often mentioned), but even more so with cosmetics. Unlike so many of us, the Beauties interviewed do not possess drawers upon drawers of eye makeup and lipsticks. They find a color they like and then they stick with what works!

EARTH COLORS ARE SAFEST FOR WOMEN WHO ARE NOT USED TO WEARING MAKEUP. BRANCH INTO COLORS GRADUALLY.

THE WRONG COLORS, ESPECIALLY COLORS THAT ARE TOO BRIGHT, FROSTED, ETC. WILL STAND OUT IN A WAY THAT IS GARISH.   IT PRESENTS A LOOK TO THE WORLD OF MIXED MESSAGES:

       A. I don't know what I'm doing.

       B. I want to be noticed, and I don't care what I have to do to achieve my goal.

       C. I suffer from a lack of confidence and need to hide behind these colors.

       D. I am a fool for fashion.

       E. I am needy.

       F. I refuse to change.

NEUTRAL AND EARTH COLORS ARE ALWAYS RIGHT BECAUSE:

       A. They give you more mileage
       B. They look richer

Real beauties impressed me with the way that they seem to get the most from their products.   For instance, they have a real knack for getting the most from their scents.

APPLY AT PULSE POINTS: ANKLES, PALMS, BACK OF KNEES, BENDS OF ELBOWS, BEHIND EARS, BASE OF THROAT, INSIDE WRISTS, UNDER TOES, AND BREASTS.

LAYER FRAGRANCE WITH MATCHING BATH AND BODY PRODUCTS.

APPLY SCENT AFTER BATH OR SHOWER WHEN PORES ARE MOST OPEN.

SPRAY SCENT INTO FRESHLY WASHED HAIR.

START LIGHTLY IN THE MORNING, AND ADD MORE AS THE DAY GOES ON. END UP WITH THE STRONGEST SCENT (PERFUME) FOR THE EVENING.

APPLY A LITTLE OF YOUR FAVORITE SCENT TO A POCKET HANKY.   PUT THE HANKY IN A POCKET ON YOUR LAPEL. ENJOYING YOUR SCENT THROUGHOUT THE DAY IS A FORM OF AROMATHERAPY.

MORE IMPORTANT ADVICE

ONCE A WEEK, LOOK AT YOURSELF IN A MAGNIFYING
MIRROR, OR EVEN BETTER, A LIGHTED MIRROR
LIKE THE ONES USED IN BACK STAGE DRESSING ROOMS.

*Remove any excess hair from upper lip, chin,
and between brows using a good pair of tweezers.*

LEARN TO WALK LIKE A MODEL FOR A TALLER,
LEANER LOOK.

*Always walk with one foot in front of the other
Pull your shoulders back
NEVER look down at the ground
Tuck in your butt
Stretch your torso*

DIP A WET TOOTHBRUSH INTO BAKING SODA
TO KEEP TEETH SPARKLING WHITE

ALWAYS USE A LOOFAH WHEN BATHING

DRINK WATER WHENEVER YOU WALK INTO A
ROOM THAT HAS ANY AVAILABLE

TIME SAVERS
Bathe or shower with scented soap
Revive a made up face with a spritz of water

THE REAL SECRETS OF BEAUTY

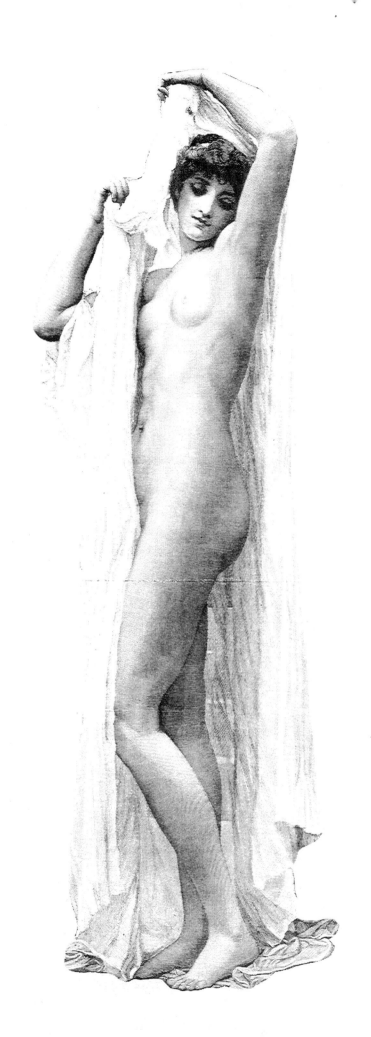

CHAPTER FIVE

SECRETS

OF

BEAUTIFUL

SKIN

MORNING ROUTINE

1. CLEANSE: It's simple. The cleansing routine of
the most beautiful women is NOT
to over scrub. Most of these women
do not use soap. If they do, it is a mild
facial soap (never a deodorant soap), but
usually it is a cleanser made especially
for their type of skin.

Dry skin?   Use a milky cleanser
Oily skin?   A clear cleanser or gel is best

2. EXFOLIATE: This is necessary to get the blood
flowing into the face and to remove surface
grime like blackheads and imbedded dirt

Pure oatmeal mixed with water is an inexpensive exfoliant
Sensitive skins should use instant oatmeal.
Some beauties use instant on their face and regular
grind on their bodies. It is especially good on
cellulite areas.

ALSO TRY:
Sugar and olive oil   **Salt and olive oil**

3. TONE: All the residue soap and exfoliant is removed
with toners and astringent
Don't waste your money on expensive cosmetic counter
toners. Here's what I found the Beauties using
(Yes, they have money for the expensive stuff)

Witch hazel   **Boric acid (in liquid form)**
Rosewater   **Lemon juice**

4. MOISTURIZE: The advice here is simple but sweet!
Don't spend a lot for a moisturizer
Do try the alpha hydroxy and glycolic acids
*buy them in drugstores
*they "unglue" top surface layers
Try to avoid mineral oil in any product

TIPS...TIPS...TIPS
HERE'S A POTPOURRI OF SKIN CARE ADVICE GATHERED FROM BEAUTIES WITH SPECTACULAR COMPLEXIONS

Vitamin E inside and out
Start the day with 1000 MG
At night break open the capsule and apply to face concentrating around the eyes.

BELIEVE IT OR NOT!

<u>Milk of Magnesia</u> straight from the bottle as a face mask

<u>Preparation "H"</u> (even I didn't believe this until I tried it) for a quick face lift. After all, if it can shrink THOSE tissues, it can shrink UNDER EYE puffiness.

<u>Kitty litter</u> and water as a face mask (do make sure that the bag indicates that it is pure clay)

<u>Bee Balm</u> A product actually used to soften cow's udders is being used as an extra strength moisturizer

<u>Mane 'n Tail</u> A horse's shampoo that several beauties with gorgeous locks claim that it leaves their hair thick, shiny, and soft

<u>Hoofmaker</u> This is a hoof conditioner that women are using to soften their hands and feet

WHY DON'T YOU TRY:

Applying a man's shaving gel to your face.
Leave it on while you shower and then rinse thoroughly.
It is a treatment that leaves the skin invigorated.

Adding sliced lemons and/or orange slices to your bath
to cleanse and refresh naturally.

Using a humidifier throughout the winter months

RECIPES RIGHT FROM NATURE

SKIN REFRESHER
Blend one cucumber with a small amount of yogurt or milk
Smooth on face and let dry.   Rinse and pat face gently

SUPER SKIN MOISTURIZER
Mash a small banana with a small amount of honey.
Pat gently on face.   Let set for about 15 minutes.

Note: There is a well known beauty who uses this recipe
on her breasts. She spreads the banana mash on
her entire breast area and then puts an old bra
on top to hold it in place. This lovely
lady claims the results are spectacular!

MORE JEWELS FOR THE SKIN

Nail brushes make the best complexion tools. You'll find them easy to handle, and the smaller size just right to get into the sides of the nose and under the jaw line.

SLEEPING BEAUTY

Try to get into the habit of sleeping on your back to prevent wrinkles. It is also helpful in preventing fluid build up around the face.

GOLDEN RULE: Always exercise without makeup

Why don't you:

Fill a pan with boiling water. Put your face over the steam for a few minutes to open your pores.

Refresh your face with chamomile tea. Put the tea in a spray bottle and keep in the refrigerator. It also aids in tightening the skin.

Muscles Sore?

Epsom Salts in the bath are effective

Foot soap is exhilarating

Also try sea salts and baking soda

SOMETIMES THE BEST THINGS IN LIFE REALLY ARE FREE!
(at least when it comes to skin care)

Ask any successful beauty. It may be trite to hear again,
but it's water that keeps that skin glowing.   In every interview
the number one secret of famous and everyday REAL beauties is
water inside and out.   No cream has the hydrating success of water.
Here's what you need to do:

DRINK 6 TO 8 GLASSES A DAY

**Yes it's boring, but worth it. Let it become a wonderful
rewarding habit by drinking whenever you think of it.**

SPRAY IT ON YOUR FACE.

**It's not necessary to spend a lot on those
"imported" water sprays. Get your own spritzer
at any beauty supply shop or use a plant spray in
a pinch.**

****

*Occasional juice fasts are popular among beautiful women to cleanse
the body and clear the skin.*

****

Wash your bangs daily to prevent an oily, broken out forehead

****

*AIR CONDITIONING IS VERY DRYING TO THE SKIN.   DRINK
LOTS OF LIQUIDS AND USE EXTRA MOISTURIZER*

VITAMINS A AND C ARE THE VITAMINS
MOST DIRECTLY RELATED TO SKIN HEALTH

Wheat germ oil is important in keeping skin elastic and in preventing stretch marks.

****

Through the ages great beauties have cleansed their face with raw honey.

****

Prone to breakouts? A five per cent solution of salicylic acid (sold in drugstores) is the perfect astringent for both morning and evening maintenance.

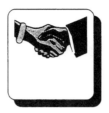

HANDS DOWN

Always purchase an acetone-free polish remover.
Removers are the source of many nail problems.

Though formaldehyde has a drying effect on nails, polish
containing small amounts tend to be longer lasting.

Puncture a vitamin E capsule and apply to cuticles at least
once a week to condition.

Stick fingers in grapefruit to whiten nails

Massage hands with cream and cover with cotton gloves.
Keep hands covered overnight for a deep penetrating
treatment.

Let fingers rest a day between manicures.
It gives them a chance to "breathe".

<u>SECRETS</u>

"I know this sounds absolutely crazy but it works.
There is a bath cleaner called "Enforcer" that
I use to exfoliate my face. The main ingredients
are citric acid and glycolic acid. These acids are
the very same as the ones in the new moisturizers.
I dilute it with water or cream. I only keep it on
a moment, but I have been absolutely startled at
the results."
JOAN, 48/ACTRESS

"Men seem to have younger looking skin because of
their many years of shaving. I recognize this as a
form of exfoliation, so I am copying these men.
Every morning I carefully shave my face!"
STEPHANIE, 40/THERAPIST

"I use Noxema to wake up my face and body. The
tingle is absolutely invigorating!"
LINDA, 35/TV PRODUCER

"Pepto-Bismol makes a great face mask."
MELANIE, 49/PROFESSOR

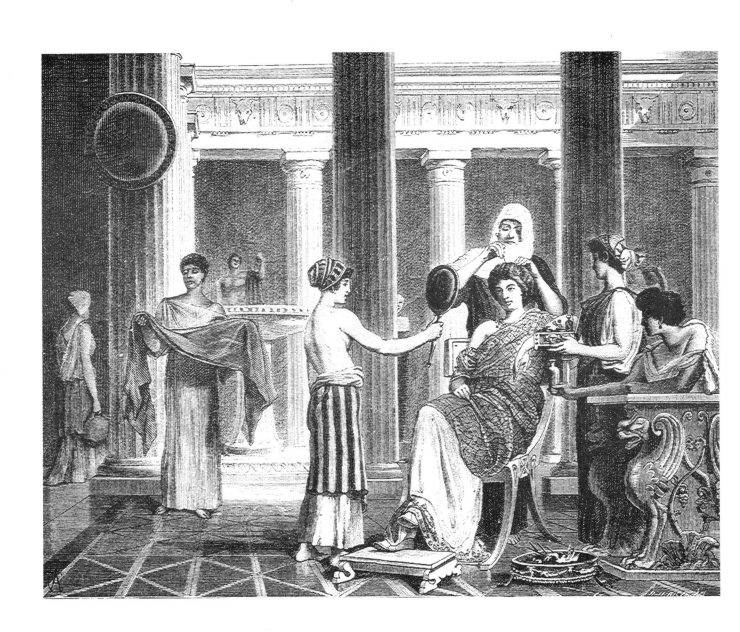

CHAPTER SIX

SECRETS

OF

MAKING UP

Always apply makeup to a clean face.
Toner will help makeup go on more smoothly

HOW TO SHOP COSMETICS COUNTERS
Take advantage of free makeovers
If the salesperson is wearing her makeup in a style or color scheme that does not appeal to you, keep going!

BASIC STEPS TO REAL BEAUTY

1. MOISTURIZE
Use a light moisturizer to wear under foundation

There are many beauties who prefer not to wear any foundation.
For them, a tinted moisturizer takes the place of step 2.

If using a glycolic or alpha-hydroxy treatment, be certain that it is in the form of a moisturizer.   Otherwise a moisturizer over this product is most necessary to counteract the strong effects.

2. FOUNDATION

Techniques for finding skin tones
* Do you look best in pure white?
You have cool undertones.

* Do you look better in cream or off white?
You have warm undertones

Take a coral lipstick and a dark pink lipstick.
Make a small stripe with each on the inside of your
wrist. If your skin more closely resembles the
coral lipstick, then your skin has yellow undertones.
If your skin more closely resembles the dark pink
lipstick, you have pink undertones.
Knowing this, you can confidently purchase
products at self service counters and drugstores.

AN EXTRA APPLICATION OF FOUNDATION
WILL ACT AS A MORE NATURAL LOOKING
CONCEALER.

APPLICATION

1. Apply with fingers or sponge

2. Start at UNDER EYE area. This is where coverage is generally most needed.

3. Blend all over face including lips.
   Sometimes you don't need to apply foundation to your entire face. If your skin is fairly flawless, then all you need to do is to cover the UNDER EYE area, spider veins, shadows, and red patches.

   *** FOUNDATION MUST MATCH SKIN PERFECTLY !***

If you are looking for a good everyday type of foundation, try to get one in a combination of foundation and powder.

ADD A LITTLE EXTRA FOUNDATION
OR CONCEALER WHERE NEEDED.

4. CONTOUR

.....Create your own illusions by using a darker
(than your skin tone) foundation by your
cheekbones, jaw line, sides of nose, etc.

*There is absolutely no need to spend big money
on expensive contouring cream. Use a foundation
2 or 3 shades darker to blend into your skin
for a more natural appearance.*

5. APPLY EYESHADOW

6. CURL LASHES

7. LINE WITH PENCIL OR LIQUID LINER

8. MASCARA

9. LIP PENCIL

......pencil outside of lips
......to really make lips stand out, pencil entire lip
......if pencil is too hard, rub between finger
to soften

10. LIPSTICK

.....make sure to blot

11. POWDER LIGHTLY

WEEKLY MAINTENANCE

TWEEZE EYEBROWS

Brush the brow upward and outward by using a small eyebrow brush so that you can see the natural line.

Tweeze from under the brow

Soften the sting by rubbing the area with an ice cube

I KNOW IT HURTS TO TWEEZE, BUT ONCE YOU GET STARTED, YOU WILL ACTUALLY "DESENSITIZE" YOUR SKIN.

TO DETERMINE WHERE TO TWEEZE

Take a pencil and put the eraser on your nostril. Where it stands straight up is where your eyebrow should start. Now direct it from the nostril to the brow bone. This is exactly where your eyebrow should end.

CLEAN OUT YOUR SKIN

Use this "laxative" for your face just like models
and actresses have done for years.

Make a tea using laxative flakes.
Steam your face for 5 to 10 minutes.

Rinse.

*You can purchase laxative flakes
at nutrition and health stores.*

*The one brand that was most
commonly mentioned as being
highly effective:*

"SWISS MISS HERBAL FLAKES"

REAL MAKEUP TIPS THAT REALLY WORK

FOUNDATION UNDER LIPSTICK HELPS IT STAY
  Forget the expensive lip fixes.   Foundation is
  as good or better.

ALWAYS FINISH LIPSTICK WITH POWDER

THERE IS NO NEED FOR MORE THAN ONE LIP PENCIL
    Neutral or brown are best bets!

**LAYER YOUR MASCARA RATHER THAN CLUMP
IT ON.**
      Your local cosmetics supply store carries an
      indispensable tool call a "lash separator".
      It is a little comb that allows you to apply more
      mascara without clumping.

**THROW AWAY THE BRUSHES THAT COME WITH
YOUR BLUSH.   THEY LEAVE AN UNNATURAL
"STRIPE" ACROSS THE FACE.**
      Use a dome shaped natural bristle brush.
      Make sure to shake brush before applying.

TIPS CONT.

SECRETS TO LIPS THAT LAST

Condition with Blistex or Chapstik

After applying lipstick pucker lips into an "O".   Cover finger in tissue and poke into mouth and twist away excess color that will eventually end on your teeth or your coffee cup.

USE ONE COLOR EXCLUSIVELY WHEN TRYING TO ACHIEVE THE "NATURAL" LOOK

SURPRISE!

Brown shadow or liner makes blue eyes bluer; green eyes greener.

Blue shadow on blue eyes and green shadow on green eyes simply looks dated!

A LITTLE BIT OF RED OR ORANGE IN THE CENTER OF THE LIPS WILL MAKE THEM LOOK FULLER

WHITE EYE SHADOW ON THE BROW BONE MAKES EYES BIGGER AND BRIGHTER.

TIPS CONT.

IF YOU FIND THAT YOUR EYELINER IS TOO HARSH OR HEAVY HANDED, SOFTEN THE LOOK WITH A SWEEP OF SHADOW CLOSE TO THE LINER COLOR.

****

POWDER MAKES BIG PORES DISAPPEAR

****

TO KEEP EYE SHADOW WORKING ALL DAY, SWEEP THE EYE WITH A BIT OF POWDER AS A BASE.

****

TO BRING OUT UPPER LIP, DAB A BIT OF HIGHLIGHTER INTO THE AREA UNDER THE NOSTRIL

TIPS CONT.

A SPRAY OF MINERAL WATER WILL RENEW A MADE UP FACE

****

TO CORRECT SEVERE FACIAL IMPERFECTIONS THAT CANNOT BE COVERED WITH TRADITIONAL MAKEUP, USE CAMOUFLAGE CREAMS SUCH AS **DERMABLEND** *OR* **LYDIA'S COVER MARK.**

****

IF YOUR FOUNDATION IS NOT IMPECCABLY MATCHED TO YOUR COMPLEXION, MAKE SURE TO BRING THE FOUNDATION LIGHTLY ON TO THE NECK AREA.

Wearing a low cut neck? Bring foundation even more lightly down to the chest area.

TIPS CONT.

NEVER DRAG A BLUSH BRUSH ON THE FACE.
1. **Use a gentle back-and-forth motion.**
2. **Have enough on the brush to be able to apply lightly.**

WASH ALL BRUSHES REGULARLY.
> **Use a mild soap**
> **Let air dry**

THROW AWAY OLD MAKE UP.
> **If you haven't used it up in 6 to 8 months you probably didn't like it that much anyway!**

DATE ALL COSMETIC PURCHASES.

SET EYELINER WITH MATCHING SHADOW.
YOU WILL FIND IT MUCH MORE EFFECTIVE THAN USING EXPENSIVE POWDER LINERS.

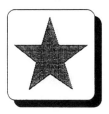

EVENING SPARKLE

Real life beauties affirm that what is acceptable as evening makeup looks cheap and tacky if worn during daylight hours.   Here are the rules of wearing make up after hours.

Everything is bolder in the evening.
> **Go with black liner and darker shadow**

Find one focal point and play it up.
> **Bright red mouth**
> **Dramatic eyes**
> **"Couture" look of deep contouring**

Heavier foundation is important.

Add gold to eyes, lips, cheeks.

Go heavier on powder. YOU want to shine; not your face.

MAKEUP MISHAPS

Sometimes makeup goes wrong. We use too heavy
a hand, or something that looked great in a magazine
has us looking like a leftover Mardi Gras queen.
Here's some help!

**GET RID OF THAT SLEEPY LOOK BY
APPLYING NAVY LINER TO TOP
LID AND MASCARA ONLY TOP LASHES.**

BLUSH ERRORS

**Wrong Placement: Smile and lightly sweep over
the apples of cheeks**

**Contouring: Blush is not a contour and you
don't blush up by your ears**

**Color: A lighter color will eliminate the
striped or clown look**

MAKE EYES WIDER BY APPLYING LIGHTER SHADOW INSIDE EYES AND JUST UNDER BROW.

BLEND.......BLEND.......BLEND

By learning to blend, makeup becomes part of the face with no lines to take away from the natural look.

TO PREVENT LINES AROUND THE EYES CAUSED BY MAKEUP FALLING INTO CREASE, PAT EYE CREAM GENTLY UNDER THE EYE AND WIPE OFF EXCESS. THEN APPLY CONCEALER OR FOUNDATION.

BRONZING POWDER IS NOT JUST FOR SUMMER. IT GIVES A MUCH MORE FLATTERING LOOK THAN TRANSLUCENT POWDER AND CAN BE USED AS A SOFT BLUSH OR CONTOUR AID.

Shadow on the lids gives a much softer look than liner and is perfect for daytime wear. As the day goes on, simply touch up with more shadow. In the evening, blend in a little pencil liner in the same color or one shade darker.

WHEN WE WORK WITH A YOUNG MODEL, WE USE
EXTREMELY HEAVY MAKEUP TO MAKE HER LOOK
OLDER AND MORE SOPHISTICATED.
THAT TELLS US THAT COSMETICS USED IN EXCESS
CAN BE QUITE AGING.

If you use too much base, it will fall into the
crevices (lines) of your face.
If you have droopy lids, you should not
use a lot of shadow.

Colors should always blend. Blue eyeshadow,
peach blush, and red lipstick on one
face SHOUT fashion victim.

Take charge of your face.   Find out what
works for you, and use it.   The approach
is to take your best look and update it through
the years.   Sophia Loren has done it, as well
as Liza Minelli, and Paloma Picasso. These
are women who have maintained their own
unique look. They haven't changed their style,
but remain elegant and up to date.

These women's faces are not perfect. They
have flaws. What makes them appear so
lovely is knowing how, with the
use of makeup, to accentuate what is great
and disguising what is not.

REAL LIFE BEAUTIES SHARE THEIR BEST MAKEUP   SECRETS

"My makeup is never complete unless I go outside in the sunlight
with a mirror.   Then I can correct heavy or not enough touches."
CASSIE, 36/MODEL

"I start my makeup lightly in the morning and layer it as the day goes on.
This helps me not only to touch up, but my coverage is perfect
for my evening out."

PATRICIA, 43/RETAILER

"My eyebrows get a lot of attention because I feel they are the
frame for my face. My eyebrow pencil is my favorite makeup
tool, and my brows are the first thing I do to my face. When my
eyebrow are made up properly, I can get away with a lot less
eye makeup."

ROSEMARY, 53/ACTRESS

"Old fashioned red rouge is my savior.   No matter how little
sleep I get or how bad I'm feeling, it always perks me up.
I buy it at the Five and Dime."

STEPHANIE, 40/ADVERTISING

"I have bought every mascara on the market, and paid up
to $20.00 a tube. Nothing beats GREAT LASH by Maybelline.
It makes my lashes huge!"

CASSANDRA,28/MODEL

"I use my blush as my lip powder, and my eye pencil as my lip
pencil".   I hate lots of "stuff".

MIMI, 39/FASHION DESIGNER

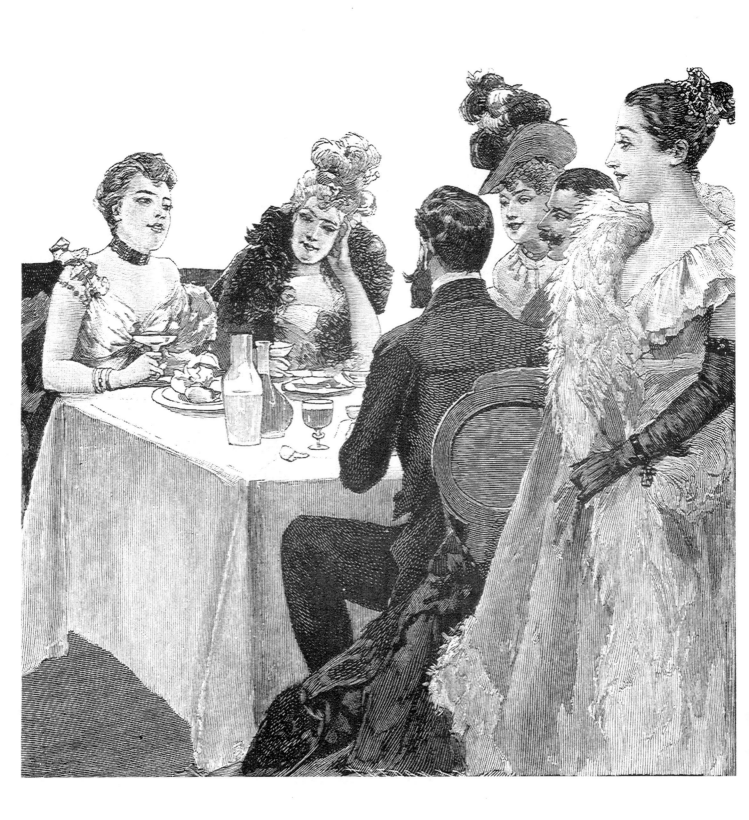

CHAPTER SEVEN

SECRETS

OF

DIETING

A diet cannot and will not work unless it consists of foods that you love.

Every diet should feature foods that are quick and easy to prepare.
Even better when meals can be prepared ahead of time!

MAKE A DAILY COMMITMENT TO DIETING BY KEEPING A FOOD DIARY.

YOUR REFRIGERATOR NEEDS A PICTURE.

You at your ideal weight
A picture from a magazine

PUT MIRRORS IN YOUR KITCHEN. IF YOU CAN STAND IT, DON'T EAT WITHOUT SITTING IN FRONT OF A MIRROR.

USE BETTER QUALITY INGREDIENTS
You'll find yourself using less.
BEST OLIVE OIL
FRESH HERBS   ETC. ETC.

What you think of as hunger, very often is thirst.
Satisfy with water or low calorie drinks. There are
wonderful flavors on the market today.   If you have
a hard time drinking plain water, add slices of lemon.
The successful dieters I interviewed reported that
using lemon achieved the same results (killing
appetite, etc.) as grapefruit.

THAT AWFUL TASTE IN YOUR MOUTH (KETOSIS)
CAN LEAD TO EATING. INSTEAD, BRUSH YOUR
TEETH AND TONGUE. A SPEARMINT, PEPPERMINT,
OR CINNAMON MOUTHWASH WILL ALSO TAKE
AWAY THAT TASTE ORDINARILY REMOVED
WITH FOOD.

Use chicken, vegetable, and beef stock instead of butter
as a sauté.   Food will taste better too!

 IF YOU DO BINGE, GET YOURSELF OUT OF   THE
REVERIE BY YELLING "STOP"
OUT LOUD, AND STANDING UP.

When you eat poultry and meat, be sure to remove
all skin and fat. Do you really want that stuff in your
body?

EAT BREAKFAST LIKE A KING
LUNCH LIKE A PRINCE
DINNER LIKE A PAUPER

WHY?

1. You'll be more active during the day and burn your calories more efficiently.

2. You will function more energetically with the proper fuel.

3. You will not be consumed with thoughts of food all day if you reach your satiety level or a reasonable level of satisfaction.

EAT PIZZA!

Just leave off the cheese.
Put as many low calorie toppings as you like.
MUSHROOMS, ONIONS, PEPPERS, ETC.

Reward yourself!
Get those earrings, flowers, manicure or other treat.

YOU DESERVE IT!

MORE TIPS:

Chew gum when cooking
Use salsa and mustard as condiments
Never eat standing up
Use small serving dishes

DRINK WATER
Before and during meals to fill up!

TRY TO COOK RIGHT AFTER MEALTIME
** Same goes for food shopping

MORE DIET DOS:
Stick to a regular eating schedule
Plan one treat a day
Eat more carbohydrates in the morning

EAT BREAD!
It is not the enemy.
Beauties report that it calms nerves and ends cravings like no other food can.

HUNGRY AT NIGHT?

Take an evening bath.
Drink a cup of tea with milk.

There are teas on the market with calming
ingredients. Look for names like "sleepy time".

Buy a full length mirror and look in it every morning
before getting dressed. **BE OBJECTIVE.**

**PICTURE THAT FATTENING FOOD AS DOING
TERRIBLE THINGS TO YOUR BODY. CONVERSELY,
THINK OF THAT APPLE, SALAD, ETC. AS RESTORING
YOUR BODY'S HEALTH AND BEAUTY.**

LET YOUR TOAST COOL BEFORE BUTTERING.
IT WILL ABSORB LESS CALORIES.

Successful dieters make fruits and vegetables the bulk of
their diet.

Cereal is usually fat-free. Occasionally substitute
lunch with cereal and toast for an under 200 calorie meal.

REAL LIFE BEAUTIES NEVER GO WITHOUT BREAKFAST.
Experts state that the most powerful of all appetite
stimulating chemicals are secreted in the morning

DINING OUT TRICK
Order hors d'oeuvres instead of entrees.

You'll find foods that are puffed, whipped, or popped
have fewer calories.

THE ONLY PEOPLE WHO BUY
DIET FOODS ARE OVERWEIGHT.

WRITE A LETTER TO YOURSELF ABOUT WHY
YOU WANT TO LOSE WEIGHT.

You need a daily serving of protein that is about
the size of your palm.

HOW TO PARTY

1. Wear your most figure revealing outfit
Don't wear anything too comfortable.
You'll be more conscious of your body.

2. Bring a delicious low calorie dish.
You'll have something you can eat..

MORE DIET ADVICE:

Diet five pounds at a time.

Eat only what you love.
There are no forbidden foods.

Make food fun again.

Don't set unrealistic weight goals.
*If you have never weighed 120 pounds, chances
are that your body is not meant to go down
to that weight.*

Learn to relax about food.
*Most women think that there are
only two ways to eat.*

BINGE

or

STARVE

MAKE A TOTAL EFFORT
1. Start your own makeover when you begin your diet.
2. Purchase one outfit in your goal size and hang it in the closet where you can see it daily.

****

When you need to munch, reach for cereal or popcorn.

****

Drink water with coffee and tea since both are dehydrating.

****

Remember that certain foods give beauty while others take it away.

****

Eat for beauty. After all, when you plant a flower don't you use the best soil?

****

Begin a meal with something fresh.

Body image makes up 30% of self esteem.

****

Sometimes you just need to nourish your soul.

****

Connect with someone rather than some food.

****

Do not try to restore your energy level with food.

****

If you aren't buying it.......then you're not eating it.

SHOP THIN!

NO MATTER HOW HUNGRY YOU ARE, WHEN YOU ARRIVE HOME WAIT AT LEAST 15 MINUTES BEFORE BEGINNING TO EAT.

****

LOVE IS A WONDERFUL APPETITE SUPPRESSANT.

****

Some spices will increase metabolism.
 They also enhance even the dullest foods.
 Start a collection.
 Experiment with foods.

****

WHATEVER YOU EAT, YOU'LL END UP WEARING.

TRIGGERS TO OVEREATING

1. TOO MUCH VARIETY
Avoid buffets
Plan meals

2. MUSIC
Avoid loud and fast music
Play soft and calming background sounds

3. DISTRACTIONS
Don't read or watch TV while eating

4. STRESS
Confront the issue if you can
Learn relaxation techniques

5. SOCIAL EVENTS
Go for the people not the plate
Find something to hold while chatting

6. FEELINGS
Don't be afraid to feel those feelings.
Stuffing it down won't take those feelings
away. It just temporarily stuffs them
down!

FIBER IS KEY TO DIETING SUCCESS.
It fills you up and keeps the system cleansed.
This is the recipe I share with my clients and friends.
It has lots of bran and is delicious and moist!

MY FAVORITE BRAN MUFFINS

2 1/2 CUPS BRAN
2 1/4 CUPS MILK OR NON FAT YOGURT
Combine and let stand until bran is absorbed.

2 EGGS
1/2 CUP SHORTENING
1 3/4 CUPS FLOUR
2 TABLESPOONS BAKING POWDER
3/4 CUP SUGAR

Combine above with bran mix.
Bake in muffin tins at 400 degrees for 10 minutes.

SECRETS

"I absolutely adore subs. There is no way in
the world that I would be able to stay slim
without having them. I make up a huge sub
sandwich with everything imaginable. I pile
on pickles, onions, lettuce, mushroom, peppers,
the works. The big secret? I leave out the
bread. It finally dawned on me that the only
fattening part of a sub is the bread. Now I
can have my sub without feeling guilty!"

Lottie, 44/Artist

"Once a week I have a day of cereal. Cereal
has virtually no fat, and I find it very filling.
It works for me!"

Cathy, 21/Model

"I buy specialty breads and incorporate them
into whatever diet I happen to be on. Bread
calms my nerves and adds variety to my diet."

Darlene, 18/Model

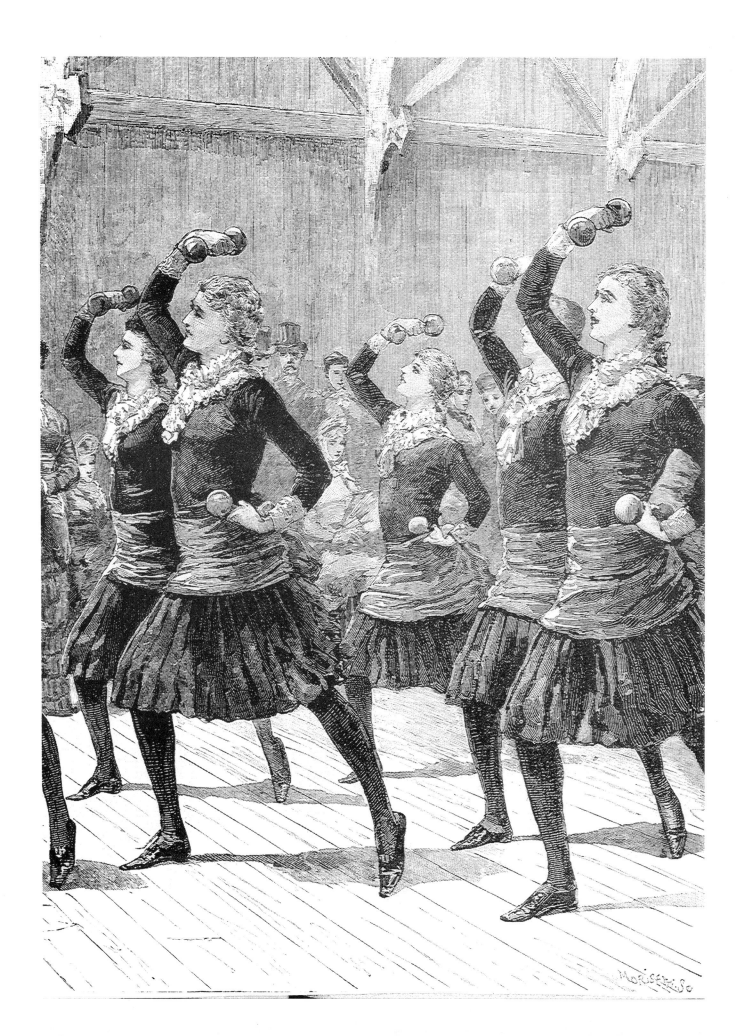

CHAPTER EIGHT

SECRETS

OF

FITNESS & HEALTH

GREAT BEAUTIES EXERCISE FOR WHAT IT DOES FOR THEIR COMPLEXION AS MUCH AS WHAT IT DOES FOR THEIR BODY.

Revs up circulation
Cleans Pores
Exfoliates skin
Removes toxins from skin

NEED TO START A FITNESS PROGRAM? DIG OUT THESE PHOTOS:
You at your very worst
You at your best
You've done it before and you can do it again.
Photo of an old beau
What if you meet again unexpectedly?

REMOVE ALL MAKEUP BEFORE EXERCISING

ACTRESSES AND MODELS LOVE THE BUTT SQUEEZE
No matter where you are, squeeze your bottom in
and out several times. Do it discreetly, please.

FOUNTAIN OF YOUTH
The Swedish Herbal Institute has come out with CHISANDRA
and ARTIC ROOT "ADAPTOGENS" (trademarked)
which are natural supplements that can re-energize cells to
look and feel younger and stronger. Check out this natural
way to turn back the clock at 1-800-774-9444.

ARE YOU FIT?

Here's one way to find out.

Walk a mile as fast as you can. The moment you finish, take your pulse. If you have walked a mile in 18 minutes with a pulse rate of 140, your cardiovascular rate is average.

****

MOVING IS EXERCISE.   HOUSEWORK AND GARDENING ARE BOTH FORMS OF EXERCISE.

****

DON'T DO ANY EXERCISE THAT YOU DON'T ENJOY. YOU WON'T STAY WITH IT, AND IT WILL LEAVE YOU WITH A BAD TASTE FOR EXERCISE IN GENERAL.

****

EVEN THE SMALLEST AMOUNT OF EXERCISE WILL GREATLY INCREASE YOUR CONFIDENCE LEVEL

****

TRY TO EAT LIGHTLY DURING EVENING HOURS. YOU'LL SLEEP BETTER AND LOSE FASTER.

ARE YOUR UNDERARMS STILL WAVING
GOOD BYE AFTER YOU HAVE LONG STOPPED?
THIS IS AN EASY TO FIX PROBLEM, AND
ALL YOU HAVE TO DO IS GRAB THE HEAVIEST
OBJECT YOU CAN COMFORTABLY LIFT.

Take the object (book, weight, soda bottle, etc.)
in your hand with arm outstretched. Bend over
and reach back and up. Do this at least 15 times.
Repeat with opposite hand. Palms must be
facing backwards.   One traveling beauty I know uses
the Gideon Bible in her hotel room for this exercise.
I must admit that her arms are quite firm!

****

GINSENG IS A NATURAL, CAFFEINE FREE BOOST.
TAKE IT AS A TEA OR IN CAPSULES. MOST
BEAUTIES REPORT THAT THEY PREFER IT TO
THE OTHER ENERGY BOOSTER, B 12.   THE
LATTER HAS THE TENDENCY TO INCREASE
APPETITE.

The latest fad among the most famous beauties of today is Colonic Irrigation.   This is nothing more than an elaborate enema. Beauties have done this for years.   The philosophy that regularity is an important key to beauty was allegedly the secret to Mae West' s lovely skin. Her weekly enema regime is now being practiced by the top models and actresses of our time.

Consequences of chronic constipation include:
DULL EYES
SALLOW, MUDDY SKIN
BAD BREATH
BLOATED APPEARANCE

A high fiber diet combined with proper exercise is a more reasonable beauty tool than costly irrigation therapies. In a world filled with processed foods, extreme dieting habits, and a sedentary style of living, it is important to be aware of this approach.

YELLOWDOCK AND NETTLE TEAS ARE GOOD
WAYS TO GET IRON INTO THE BODY.

****

SEAWEED WILL BOOST A SLUGGISH THYROID.

****

VISIT YOUR CLOSEST CHINATOWN. THEIR HERB
MARKETS HAVE MANY INEXPENSIVE HERBS AND
TREATMENTS. THEIR PRICES ARE MUCH BETTER
THAN HIGH PRICED NUTRITION CENTERS.

****

TO RELIEVE TENSION OR ANXIETY MANY FAMOUS
BEAUTIES RELY ON VALERIAN EXTRACT IN
WATER. TRY FIVE DROPS. WORK UP TO NO
MORE THAN TWELVE DROPS IF NECESSARY.

****

LINDENFLOWER TEA IS GREAT FOR INSOMNIA.

PARSLEY TEA DETOXIFIES THE BODY.

CHROMIUM PICOLINATE

This supplement is a secret hunger fighter!
Not only does it turn off hunger signals.
but it boosts metabolism. 200 MG is
the recommended dose.

VITAMIN C

This beauty aid produces a skin-plumping
collagen.

VITAMIN A

Take this to regulate skin hydration and
to repair skin and nails.

VITAMIN B

This important vitamin keeps skin smooth,
promotes hair and nail growth , and
improves circulation.

VITAMIN E

Known as the skin vitamin, it has
properties to heal scar tissue and to
neutralize damaging free radicals.

Eat apples.   They contain acids that dissolve
age spots and wrinkles.

****

Use Indian Husks tea to correct irregularity.

****

Gingko Biloba is the anti-aging supplement.
From the oldest living tree, it aids in
circulation and memory.

****

Just a half hour of walking a day will
expend 1,000 calories per week. That's
an entire day of healthy eating!

****

Nikki Haskell's "Star Caps" are a natural
garlic/papaya supplement that models/actresses
are using to take away water weight.
WARNING: Stay close to a bathroom!

EXERCISE AND FITNESS TIPS OF REAL LIFE BEAUTIES

"I hate to exercise, so I do things that keep me in shape without making me get into any kind of program. I walk up stairs instead of taking elevators, I park as far away from my destination as comfortable, and I just move as often as possible."

Molly, 32/Homemaker

"Remember all the energy we had when we danced to OUR music? I put on my old records, and suddenly I can exercise for at least an hour and not even realize it. The funny thing is, I even remember some of the old steps!"

Sandy, 45/Sales & Marketing

"With all the evidence about the benefits of anti-oxidants, I make certain that I alternate extra C and E as daily supplements in my diet."

Suzanne, 50/Retail Sales

"I have made a pledge to myself that I will not watch my favorite programs without being on my stair stepper. I made this promise a year ago, and have lost 30 pounds!"

Jan, 29/Attorney

SECRETS CONT.

" I sit at a desk all day and use it to exercise my arms.
I stand by my desk and place my hands by the edge,
about a yard apart, with my palms down. Leaning
forward, I bend my elbows and lower my body until
it is parallel to the desk. Then I slowly raise my body
to my starting position.   I repeat this exercise about
15 times. It's like a mini push-up."

Sara, 35/Travel Agent

"I take this Protein punch 3 times a day. It's a youth
tonic that also controls my appetite and gives me
extra energy."

                    3 tablespoons of unflavored gelatin
                    1 banana
                    1 cup soy milk
Blend thoroughly and drink slowly.

Jenny, 47/Radio Sales

"Acupuncture is my way of staving off a face lift.
I have it done once a week, and find it relaxing
as well as beneficial."

Mary, 53/Teacher

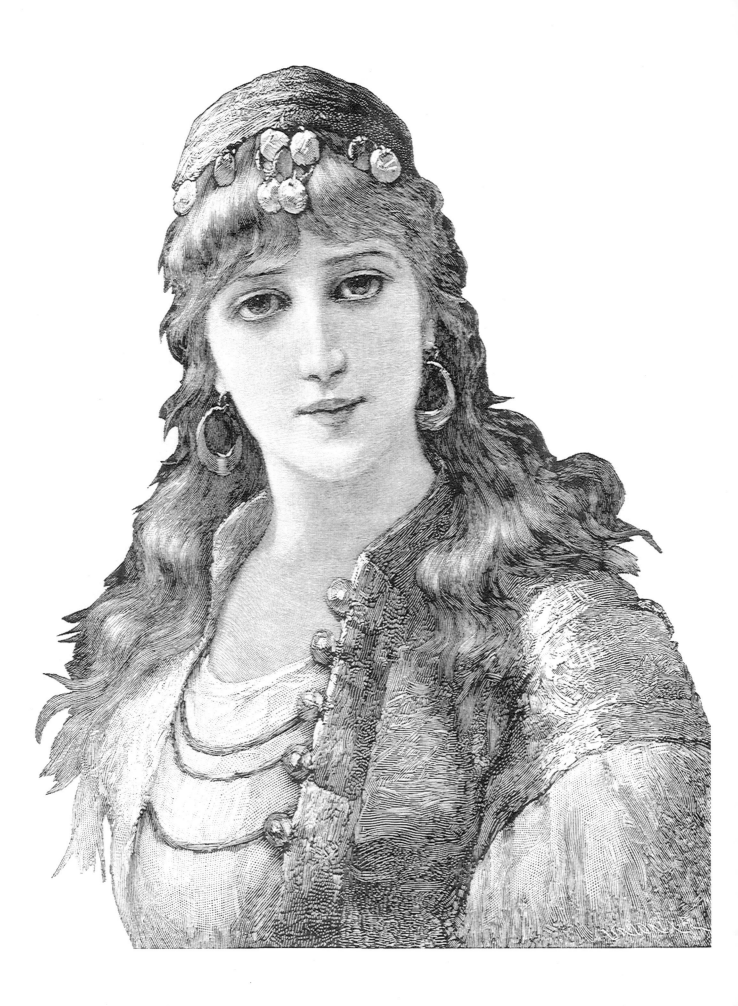

CHAPTER NINE

SECRETS
OF
BEAUTIFUL

HAIR

Your hair is undoubtedly your biggest asset when it comes to beauty. It's. look and condition can literally make or break your appearance. There are as many tips as there are beauty products. Enjoy and use each one when you are doing your own hair. Teach your hairstylist a few of them, and if there is one tip that stands above the rest it is:

FIND A STYLIST YOU LIKE AND CAN TRUST WITH YOUR HAIR.

****

A GOOD STYLIST WILL TAKE AT LEAST 30 MINUTES ON A NEW STYLE.

****

IF YOUR HAIRSTYLIST HAS HIS OWN IDEAS ABOUT HOW YOU SHOULD LOOK, INSIST THAT YOU BE SHOWN A PICTURE.

****

TAKE A PICTURE WITH YOU OF EXACTLY THE CUT THAT YOU WANT. YOU CANNOT POSSIBLY DESCRIBE WHAT A PICTURE CAN SHOW.

IT'S A PROVEN FACT! SUCCESSFUL BEAUTIES HAVE LESS HAIR DISASTERS BECAUSE THEY ENTER A HAIR SALON WITH A SPECIFIC GAME PLAN.

****

A LITTLE LEMON JUICE MIXED WITH THE FINAL RINSE OF A SHAMPOO TREATMENT ADDS SOFT HIGHLIGHTS.

****

Frizzy hair means that not enough water is in the hair shaft. Use a gloss (there are dozens on the market) to give hair a finish and to tame hair down to a silky consistency.

****

IF HAIR LOOKS FRIZZY AFTER BLOW DRYING, MIST A BRUSH WITH "LEAVE-IN" CONDITIONER. RUN THE BRUSH ALL OVER HAIR

****

Always shake head when using hairspray. This will give hair good control without weighing it down.

****

LOW FOREHEAD? LOOK FOR A STYLE WITH LONG BANGS STARTING A LITTLE HIGHER ON THE HEAD THAN USUAL. THE SAME HOLDS TRUE FOR HEADS WITH PESKY COWLICKS.

SECRETS TO BLOW DRYING

1. Start with roots and dry away from face.
2. Blow dry with fingers until almost dry.
3. Lean over and blow dry hair upside down.
4. Finish with roller brushes sized according to hair length.

SECRETS TO A GOOD STYLIST

Your stylist should ask questions.
Otherwise you'll end up with the "style of the day"

Your stylist should touch your hair when it's dry.

You should be shown pictures.

Your stylist should show you how to adapt the style and add versatility.

Your stylist must listen to your needs.
Tell her how much time you are willing to spend on your hair.

You should be able to duplicate your salon look.

Your stylist should explain what she has done.
AND WHY!!

Does your hair need a pick up? Have you gone
a little too heavy on your conditioner?
**BRUSH SOME CORNSTARCH
OR BAKING SODA THROUGHOUT.**

****

BEST HOME CONDITIONER
Blend 2 eggs with 1/2 cup olive oil
Leave on 30 minutes
Rinse thoroughly

****

TO REMOVE RESIDUE BUILD UP
Apply vinegar after shampoo
Dilute to suit
Use club soda straight from the bottle

****

USE A WIDE TOOTHED COMB ON WET HAIR
Also removes dead skin cells from scalp

USE A SPRITZ OF WATER
Refreshes style and gives an instant lift
Revitalizes gel or spray
* without adding build up

BE SURE TO SWITCH SHAMPOOS OCCASIONALLY
One brand washes away the other's residue

ADD BEER TO SHAMPOO
Adds extra shine
Removes residue

FINGER COMB HAIR WHENEVER POSSIBLE
Wet or Dry

HAIR DESERVES DRESSING UP TOO!
Use hair accessories when possible.

GROWING A STYLE OUT

1. BANGS

Spritz with gel or mousse and roll hair back or forward as length dictates

2. LAYERS

Have length cut a little shorter than usual
Invest in a soft body wave

****

ROLL AGAINST HAIR'S PATTERN FOR VOLUME

****

IF YOU'RE GROWING OUT A LAYERED CUT, IT IS NECESSARY FOR YOUR STYLIST TO CUT THE ENDS OF THE LAYERS.

To prevent split ends
Create a smoother look

CAN'T DO A THING WITH THAT HAIR AND NO TIME TO START OVER?
>Wet it and comb back with some gel
>Add a hair accessory to focus away from style

****

DON'T BRUSH HAIR MORE THAN NECESSARY.
It really doesn't do much more than spread oil around.

****

CHANGE YOUR PART OCCASIONALLY TO ADD LIFT AT THE ROOT AREA.

****

SPRAY A CUP OF STRONG CHAMOMILE TEA ON DRY HAIR AND RINSE.
>*Enhances color to blonde and brown hair*

****

SPRAY A CUP OF STRONG COFFEE ON DRY HAIR TO ADD SPARKLE TO BLACK /DARK BROWN HAIR.   RINSE THOROUGHLY.

**COLORING PROCEDURES ARE MUCH MORE
EFFECTIVE ON HAIR THAT IS DEVOID OF
SPRAYS, GELS, ETC.**

****

AVOID HAIR PRODUCTS THAT CONTAIN ALCOHOL

****

**GETTING THE URGE TO CHANGE THAT
HAIRSTYLE?**
    **Head to the nearest wig shop and try "on"
some styles first.**

****

**WHEN POSSIBLE, PLAN SHAMPOOING SO THAT
YOU CAN LET HAIR AIR-DRY UNTIL BARELY DAMP**
Limits time hair is stressed by heating tools

****

PAT HAIR (DON'T RUB) TO TOWEL DRY.

REAL LIFE SECRETS

"Once a month I use a deep conditioner on my hair and keep it on overnight. I use a shower cap to keep it in place."

                                            MELISSA, 25/MODEL

"I can make my set last days longer by sleeping on a satin pillow. I do a lot of business traveling and always bring my pillow cover with me."

                                            TAMMY, 37/SALES

"Whenever I go to the beach, I make sure that I slather my hair with conditioner. Not only am I protecting my hair from the harmful sun rays, but the sun acts as a heating lamp for the conditioner."

                                            SALLY, 19/MODEL

"Each morning and night, I rub my facial moisturizer in my hair after working on my face."

                                            VICKI, 48/FORMER MODEL

"Whenever I'm out in the sun, I use a little sun block on my hair part."

                                            PAM, 24/HAIRSTYLIST

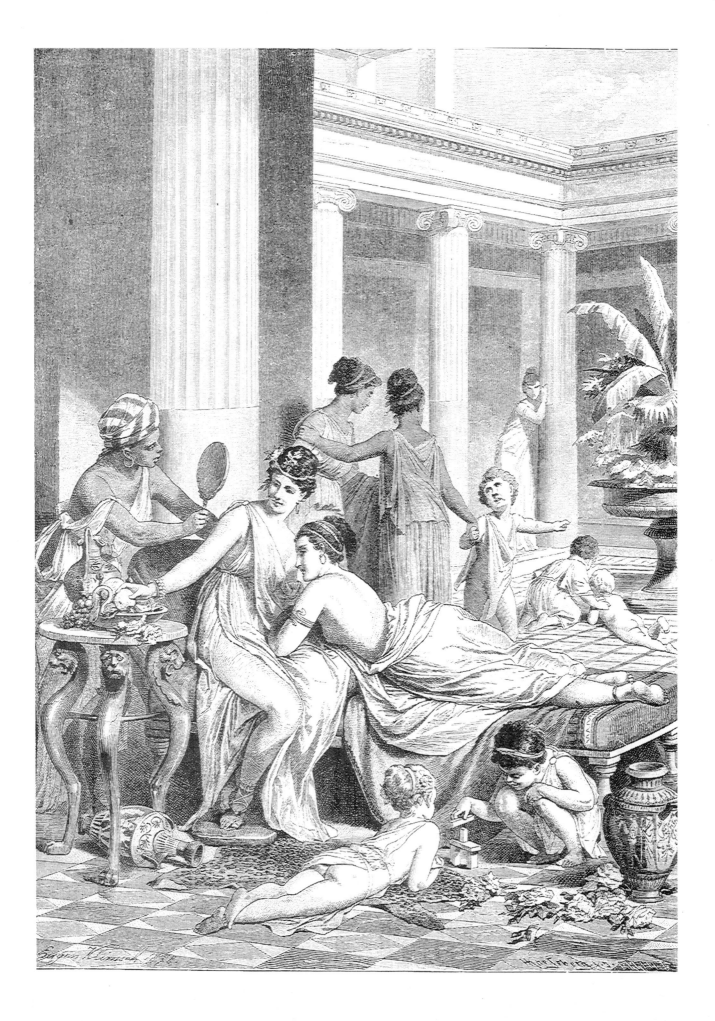

CHAPTER TEN

SECRETS

OF

STAYING

YOUNG

AGING BEAUTIES NEED TO MAKE THESE PURCHASES TO KEEP THEIR LOOKS IN CHECK.

1. THREE WAY MIRROR
This is a must to insure that you look
as good GOING as you do coming.
Some of the first signs of aging occur
from behind.

2. MAGNIFYING MIRROR
Preferably, a magnifying cosmetics mirror
to free hands, but this purchase is
essential to check on age spots, facial hair, etc.

****

MAGAZINES APPROPRIATE TO AGE
Quite frankly, some of the high
fashion magazines are too far
fetched and will only discourage
the aging beauty.

GET STARTED WITH A FRUIT ACIDS PROGRAM.
ALSO CALLED ALPHA HYDROXY ACIDS (AHA),
THESE MINI SKIN "PEELERS" WILL SLOUGH
AWAY THE LEATHERY LAYERS OF THE YEARS.

Check the percentage of acid in each
product. Get the highest percentage
your skin will tolerate.

LOOK FOR 6 TO 10 PER CENT

****

SKIN COLOR IS LOST AS WE AGE. THAT'S WHY
IT IS NECESSARY TO ADD COLOR TO THE FACE
WITH COSMETICS.

Colors that are too light or too dark
only emphasis aging features.

LEAVE THE PASTELS TO THE NURSERY.
It's a cinch to put back the "blush of youth"
into your wardrobe with lots of reds, purples,
browns, and primary color combinations.

****

AVOID FROSTED ANYTHING
That means lipstick, blush, and eyeshadow.
There is nothing more aging and dating.

****

**TRY TO AVOID FACE POWDER, AND GET A
MORE NATURAL LOOK WITH CREAM POWDER
MAKEUP. IT GOES ON LIKE A REGULAR CREAM
FOUNDATION, BUT FINISHES TO A POWDER
CONSISTENCY. IT ELIMINATES THE AGING
EFFECTS OF HEAVY POWDER WHICH
ACCENTUATES WRINKLES.**

****

ALWAYS LINE LIPS
Prevents bleeding on to surrounding wrinkles
Makes shrinking lips appear larger

**AGING BEAUTIES LEAVE BEHIND SOAPS
AND USE GELS AND CREAMS TO CLEANSE.**

****

**GINGKO BILOBA IS A SUPPLEMENT WITH
ANTI-AGING BENEFITS.**
> **Boosts blood flow**
> **Flushes away wastes that contribute
> to a sallow complexion**

****

LOOK YOUNGER TRICKS
> **Step up skin care**
> **Use less makeup**
> **Color hair**
> **Get a new hair cut**
> **Exercise**
> **Make careful clothing choices**

****

**USE NAIL POLISH EVEN IF NAILS ARE SHORT.
IT WILL TAKE ATTENTION AWAY
FROM AGE SPOTS AND VEINS.**

ANTI-AGING FOODS

Cereals	Fruits
Fish	Garlic
Yogurt	Leafy vegetables

****

COUNT FAT GRAMS
EACH GRAM OF FAT = NINE CALORIES

****

COLORED CONTACT LENSES GIVE A SPARKLE
TO THE EYES THAT IN TURN GIVE A YOUTHFUL
SPARKLE TO THE FACE.

****

GET TEETH PROFESSIONALLY CLEANED
MORE OFTEN.

****

DRESSING TOO YOUNG CAN BE AGING.

AS WE AGE, THINNER IS NOT NECESSARILY MORE ATTRACTIVE. REMEMBER THE CLASSIC FRENCH SLOGAN:
"After 40 a woman must choose between her face and her figure."

****

BLUSHING IS NOT JUST FOR CHEEKBONES.
Use it on temples, chin, and brow bone.

****

AGING BRINGS KNOWLEDGE THAT LIFE IS NOT PERFECT AND NEITHER ARE WE.

****

DO YOU PASS THE PENCIL TEST?
Here is an informal "check" to see how well you are aging from "behind"!
IF YOU CAN HOLD A PENCIL BETWEEN YOUR THIGH AND "CHEEK"...........
SORRY, YOU FAIL!

PROTECT YOUR SKIN FROM THE SUN
All of your skin
Don't forget your scalp

****

TAKE GOOD CARE OF YOUR HANDS.
They are a real age indicator.

****

FOOL THE CAMERA
When it's time to have your picture taken,
smile like you have a fish hook hanging on
each side of your mouth
(This is a secret of aging actresses/models to diminish
laugh lines and crinkles)

****

**CHANGE SHAMPOO AS YOU AGE. YOU HAVE
LESS OIL IN YOUR HAIR. DETERGENT
SHAMPOOS ARE MUCH TOO STRONG.**

A SCARF IS A GOOD WAY TO DISGUISE A CREPEY NECK.

****

SHOULDER PADS LIFT A STOOPED POSTURE.

****

SOFT PLEATS FLATTEN A TUMMY BULGE

****

ALWAYS PULL UP YOUR BRA STRAPS AND CHOOSE A BRA WITH BUILT-IN SUPPORT.

****

CONTROL TOP PANTYHOSE GIVE A SMOOTH PROFILE AND FLATTER EVERY FIGURE TYPE.

****

COLORED HOSE AND OPAQUES CAMOUFLAGE VARICOSE VEINS AND DISCOLORATIONS.

STAY AWAY FROM FADS IN FASHION, MAKEUP,
AND HAIR. CLASSIC AND UNDERSTATED
IS SAFEST FOR THE AGING BEAUTY.

****

CHECK HEMLINES.   IN-BETWEEN LENGTHS
ARE AGING.
****

CLOTHES SHOULD FIT PROPERLY. TOO LOOSE
OR TOO TIGHT IS AGING.
*GET A GOOD SEAMSTRESS AND
RELY ON HER.*

****

DEFINE YOUR BROWS FOR AN INSTANT FACE-LIFT.

****

PURE BLACK OR PURE WHITE NEAR THE FACE
NEEDS TO HAVE A BRIGHT COLOR ACCENT.

A LITTLE LONGER SLEEVE LENGTH IS MORE
FLATTERING. STAY AWAY FROM SLEEVELESS.

****

UPDATE YOUR FRAMES IF YOU WEAR GLASSES.

****

LOSE THE LACE AND PETER PAN COLLARS! IT JUST LOOKS <u>SILLY.</u>

****

CONTRARY TO WHAT YOU'VE HEARD,
LONG HAIR CAN BE QUITE LOVELY AND
FEMININE ON AGING BEAUTIES.
But DON'T wear it in a bun!

****

RELY ON PRODUCTS THAT ADDS VOLUME TO HAIR.

****

LOOSEN YOUR HAIR. SET HAIRSTYLES ARE AGING.

DON'T BECOME A CARICATURE OF WHAT
YOU WERE AT 20.   OR 30.
> Women who are guilty of this, tend to wear
> the look that they had when they were happiest,
> or when they felt most attractive.

****

GO BRIGHTER AND LIGHTER AS YOU AGE.

****

AGING BEAUTIES SHOULD DIET SLOWLY.
> Skin cannot retract as quickly.

****

GO LIGHTLY ON ALCOHOL.
> It puffs up and temporarily stretches the skin.

****

ALWAYS CURL EYELASHES
> Can't beat the way it opens the eye!

STAND TALL AND THROW SHOULDERS BACK
Appearing "bent over" adds years to the body

****

USE A COSMETIC SPONGE TO APPLY POWDER
A sponge glides over crevices and lines

****

TOO MUCH CONCEALER CAN ACCENTUATE LINES
Thin with foundation or moisturizer

****

DON'T OVER PLUCK EYEBROWS
Brows provide balance to the face

****

ACCENTUATE TOP LASHES
It takes emphasis away from laugh lines

REAL SECRETS

"To combat the increasing thinness of my aging hair,
I have invested in hair extensions. Lots of hair
is youthful!"

RITA, 56/ACTRESS

"Every so often when I am feeling "OLD", I run
to the magazine counter and grab up the ones
dedicated to the youth market. Keeping up on trends
and investing in one occasionally make me more
aware and not so "out of it."

GERRI, 48/AT HOME

"I got rid of the curls and went to straight hair.
It made me look 20 years younger!"

CHRIS, 51/PEDIATRICAN

"I use bronzer all over my face. It gives me that
well-rested look."

DIANE, 46/STOCKBROKER

"I lightened my hair and people thought I had
snuck out for a face lift."

GLORIA, 53/AT HOME

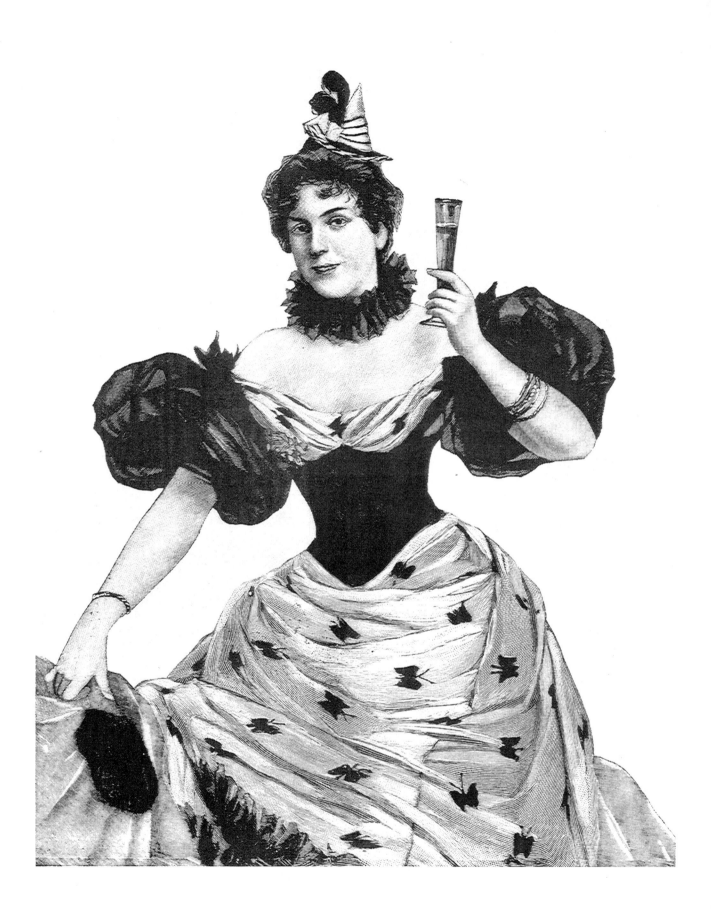

CHAPTER ELEVEN

SECRETS

OF

FASHION & STYLE

**THE SECRET TO BEING WELL-DRESSED
IS UNDER DRESSING.**

****

**USE CLASSIC PIECES AS THE BACKBONE
OF YOUR WARDROBE. THESE PIECES WILL
LAST FROM SEASON TO SEASON.**
Accessories are an inexpensive updater.

****

NEVER BLINDLY FOLLOW FASHION
You will never be fashionable unless YOU
establish the style rules.

****

**GO SHOPPING BY YOURSELF. KEEP TO YOURSELF.
FRIENDS CAN TALK YOU INTO PURCHASES
EVEN MORE PERSUASIVELY THAN SALESPEOPLE.
SIMPLY INFORM PUSHY SALES STAFF THAT YOU
PREFER SOME TIME ALONE TO CONSIDER YOUR
WARDROBE NEEDS. REMEMBER, YOU ARE
YOUR OWN BEST JUDGE.**

FIND A COAT OR SWEATER WITH AT LEAST 20% CASHMERE IN IT. YOU GET THE LOOK AND FEEL OF CASHMERE WITHOUT THE HIGH COST.

****

STAY CLEAR OF TOO MANY DETAILS IN A MAJOR PURCHASE LIKE A COAT OR JACKET.
It will stay in style a lot longer.

****

HIGH WAISTED PANTS THAT TAPER TO THE ANKLE GIVE A SLIMMING EFFECT.

****

CLASSIC PLEATED TROUSERS ARE TIMELESS AND HIDE BULGES.

****

PETITE WOMEN SHOULD AVOID FULL PANTS.
Too overwhelming to the body

****

THE LONGER THE PANT, THE LEANER THE LOOK!

**WIDE LEG PANT STYLES ARE GREAT FOR
FULL THIGHS.**

****

HOW TO WEAR MENSWEAR
"Cross Dressing" is cheap and chic!
Choose one or two pieces at a time.
STEAL: His hat, vest, leather jacket, sweater.

****

**IF YOU'RE LOOKING FOR REAL LIFE FASHION,
AVOID HIGH FASHION MAGAZINES. INSTEAD,
SEND AWAY FOR A FEW MAIL ORDER CATALOGS.**

****

SWIMSUIT SHOPPING
**SLIM A THICK WAIST WITH VERTICAL STRIPES.
SMALLER BUSTS NEED A STRUCTURED BRA.
ELONGATE THIGHS WITH HIGH CUT LEGS.
HORIZONTAL STRIPES SHORTEN A LONG TORSO.**

****

FASHION IS NOT!!!!
Looking perfect
Looking forced

SHOULDER PADS
   Makes clothes look more expensive
   Improves posture
   Brings emphasis to face
   Adds a slimming effect to body line

*****

Don't pass up that buy just because it doesn't fit perfectly.   A tailor can give that item a custom look. The very same goes for the clothes hanging in the back of your closet.

*****

BAGGY IS NEVER STYLISH

*****

DON'T LET ACCESSORIES WEAR YOU!
   If in doubt, always remove one piece

*****

NEVER BUY CLOTHES BY THE SEASON.
   There are now wools on the market that are so light that they can even be worn on the hottest summer day.

DRESSING THINNER

No matter where I am speaking, the number one
question asked is "How can I dress to look slimmer?"
Here are the rules:

1.   MATCH YOUR HOSE TO YOUR SHOES

2.   YOU CAN WEAR PRINTS, JUST PICK
     UP THE DARKEST COLOR IN YOUR
     PRINT AND BRING IT TO YOUR SHOES
     AND HOSE COLOR.

3.   FABRICS SHOULD FLOAT OVER THE
     BODY RATHER THAN CLING

******

PURCHASE THE BEST PURSE AND SHOES THAT
YOU CAN AFFORD. THEY ARE YOUR MOST
IMPORTANT ACCESSORIES. ALTHOUGH THEY
DO NOT HAVE TO MATCH, THEY SHOULD BLEND.

******

PLEASE DO NOT OVER LADEN YOUR HANDBAG.
     It's impossible to look chic with a stuffed purse
     A bad back is not a fashion statement

BARE LEGS ARE NEVER ACCEPTABLE
    Except as weekend wear

****

FASHION MISTAKE OF LARGE BUSTED WOMEN
    Carrying a handbag that is too large
    Or a purse that is too small
    Choose a bag appropriate to body proportion

****

SHORT-WAISTED WOMEN CAN EASILY WEAR BELTS. JUST ANGLE DOWN ON THE WAIST TO CREATE THE ILLUSION OF A LONGER LINE.

****

SHOPPING LINGO

    IRREGULAR: A slight flaw, generally not discernible
            to the eye

    SECOND: A major seam defect or stain. Examine carefully.

SHOES

Measure shoe size periodically. Shoe size is affected by:
   Weight gain or loss
   Aging
   Pregnancy

****

Women who are on their feet much of the day who can't live without their heels should go up at least half a size to allow for comfort and swelling.

****

MOST REALISTIC COMFORT LEVEL FOR HEELS
TWO INCHES OR LOWER

****

NEVER BUY VINYL SHOES.
They never last, and your feet can't breathe.

****

SHOES TOO TIGHT? WET INSIDE OF SHOES WITH AN EQUAL AMOUNT OF WATER AND ALCOHOL. STUFF WITH NEWSPAPER AND LEAVE OVERNIGHT.

LARGE BEAUTIES THINK
GENTLE DEFINITION
LONG OVER SHORT
LONG OVER LEAN
SAME COLOR HEAD TO TOE
ACCESSORIES THAT FRAME FACE
KNITS THAT NEVER BIND

NO ONE CAN WEAR BIG BOLD JEWELRY BETTER
No mosquito "bites" on the ear, please!

****

AT HOME DRESSING TIPS
Never let your fashion guard down even at home.
Substitute spandex for polyester.
* Keeps it shape and flatters figure
Throw away all but one "painting" outfit.
* How much painting do you really do?
At home should be easy care. Buy wash & wear.
* Look for acrylic blends
Forget sweatshirts. Buy cotton sweaters instead.
Sneakers are only for exercise.
* Choose ballet flats or loafers for comfort

WHAT TO WEAR TO THAT WEDDING?
          Dress and Jacket
          Simple dress with dazzling accessories
          Sequin top with flowing pant
          Embellished suit

******

ACCESSORIES BECOME MORE IMPORTANT WHEN THE ECONOMY GOES DOWN.

******

IF YOU LIKE WHAT YOU WEAR IT WILL SHOW ON YOUR FACE.

****

WHAT TO WEAR ON "FAT" DAYS
          Oversized blazer
          Easy waistband
          Simple sheath
          One basic color

SECRETS OF HANDBAGS

Real beauties are on the go today. To be well groomed
it is necessary to have a handbag of essentials.
A fashionable handbag is never more than 10 x 13 inches.
However, it is difficult to get all essentials into a bag
of this size. Here is a guide for the well groomed/well
organized beauty.

LIPSTICK (CAN DOUBLE AS BLUSH)
COMPACT WITH OIL CONTROL PRESSED POWDER
NOTEBOOK & PEN
ONE CHECK
COMPACT WALLET
NEUTRAL EYE SHADOW
BREATH DROPS
COMB OR BRUSH
HAIR ELASTIC
NAIL FILE
EYE PENCIL/CRAYON
MASCARA
SEWING KIT
TISSUES
MINI PILL BOX WITH EMERGENCY ASPIRIN, ETC.

Try to get sample sizes for some of above.

SECRETS OF GROOMING

The difference between being dressed and well dressed is many times that minor detail that can so easily be overlooked.

REPLACE HEELS WHEN THEY WEAR OUT
PLUCK EYEBROWS ON A REGULAR BASIS
HAVE CLOTHES CLEANED AND PRESSED
CHECK AND DOUBLE CHECK MAKEUP
REMOVE ALL FACIAL HAIR
KEEP NAILS IMPECCABLY GROOMED

****

WHAT BLACK DOES:
>   Gets you dressed that much quicker
>   Makes you look thin on "fat" days
>   Coordinates with almost anything

****

SECRETS OF PURCHASING A JACKET
>   Full figures: choose gentle draping
>   Petites: shorter length/vertical lines
>   Thin or small busted types: double breasted
>   horizontal designs

SECRETS OF SHOPPING

Begin your shopping trip in your very own closet. Split up outfits and make notes.

****

When choosing color, forget the charts. You can
wear any color that appeals to you. Just make
sure that your most visible color is your most flattering.

****

CAN'T LIVE WITHOUT CLASSICS
Pleated trousers just like Katherine Hepburn
The great white shirt (slightly oversized)
Scarves (start a collection)
Navy blazer
Aviator sunglasses

****

RULES FOR BUYING A LONG SKIRT
Tops should be snug
Keep waistline evident
Top with a fitted jacket

WORK STRATEGIES

To be successful in any business it is first necessary
to appear to be part of a team. There is of course, an
image, a projection, that is unique to every industry.
Being aware of one's image in the workplace will
insure success at every level.

It's details that count in the corporate climb. No
matter what you put on your back, it is the total
picture that makes or breaks that look. Frayed
cuffs, scuffed shoes, unkempt fingernails, messy
hair, all create an unfortunate indelible signature.

Sometimes in the very competitive workplace you
can be hired (or not) in a matter of minutes. The
look of today is polished but understated. It is
without doubt, the safest look to wear to that first
interview when you've not had an opportunity to
research the dress code.

Dress to the level of job aspiration.   For instance, if
you want to get to that senior management position, see
what the current managers are wearing. It will be too
obvious to copy an exact style, but there are key
characteristics that will become obvious.

Fashion really does matter in the business world. Clothes
communicate a message. Send the right message. Plan
your looks and wardrobe with the same care you give your
resume.

TO GET FROM WORK TO EVENING

Wear a basic skirt or slack outfit. Carry and change top, shoe, and accessories.

FASHION DON'TS!!

These fashion blunders do not apply to this year or next year. These are mistakes that have never looked fashionable and never will.

FISHNET STOCKINGS
RODEO CLOTHES
  Fringed anything
  Cowboy boots worn outside pants
SWEATSHIRTS
  Except for exercising
TIGHT KNITS
SEE-THROUGH SHOES WITH HOSE
TOO MUCH PERFUME
SOCKS WITH NYLONS
PANTY LINES
SEQUINS IN DAYLIGHT
WEARING UNDERWEAR AS CLOTHING

SECRETS OF DRESSING FOR A DIET

Clothing that is too loose can appear frumpy.
Adding a belt will help pull a look together,

Purchase one pair of leggings and wear them with
all of those loose tops and jackets.

Very loose pants can be belted for the "paper bag"
effect, but only if paired with form fitting tops.

Add extra shoulder pads to give structure to loose tops.

STAY AWAY FROM:
  Stiff fabrics
  Big pockets
  Anything ending at the body's widest part

****

*NAVY IS A COLOR THAT SEEMS TO LOOK
BEST ON EVERYONE. IT GIVES POWER
WITHOUT THE STARK UNFRIENDLINESS
OF BLACK. IT ALSO STAYS CLEAN !*

SECRETS OF SCENT
Compare price when shopping for scent.
Perfume is strongest.
Eau de parfum is next.
Third is toilet water.
Least potent is cologne.

****

LEGGINGS
Anyone can wear leggings. The secret is the more
toned the leg, the more of the legging is revealed.
Stay away from thin dance/exercise tights that
can show every imperfection.

****

ONLY A FULL LENGTH MIRROR WILL TELL YOU
IF AN OUTFIT IS WORKING IN ITS ENTIRETY.
YOU MUST OWN AT LEAST ONE. IF IT'S IN THE
BUDGET, INVEST IN A THREE WAY MIRROR.
THEY ARE AVAILABLE AT RETAIL SURPLUS SHOPS.

The best dressed beauties never make a purchase without
viewing themselves in an angled mirror. They know that it
is as important to look good going as it is coming.

Fringe that outdated short skirt with fabric trim.
  Use a hot glue gun and appliqué sequins on old handbags.
  Take old hats and decorate them with pins and brooches.
  A silk pocket square makes a funky watch strap.
  Earrings double as jewelry pins.
  Update an old jacket with new buttons.
  Old V-neck sweaters can be worn backwards in the evening.
  Update pendants with ribbon and cording.
  Shrink an oversized sweater for a new look.

****

GET TWO LOOKS FROM ONE SUIT
  Wear it with a tee shirt during the day
  Adorn it with lace at night

****

ALWAYS BUY QUALITY OVER QUANTITY

****

DRESS UP A JACKET OR COAT WITH A SHAWL
  Very European

****

GIVE A FEMININE TOUCH TO STRUCTURED SUITS
Add lace, ruffles, and bows for a new look.

FASHION MAINTENANCE

CLOTHES SHOULD AIR AFTER EACH WEARING
TO DISCOURAGE MILDEW

BRUSH CLOTHES WITH A LINT BRUSH
BEFORE HANGING

DON'T DRY CLEAN AFTER EVERY WEARING.
MOST GARMENTS CAN ONLY TAKE 20 TO
25 CLEANINGS.

NEVER LET STAINS SET. ALWAYS HAVE A
STAIN REMOVAL LOTION ON HAND.

WHEN LEATHER GETS WET, STUFF WITH
NEWSPAPERS TO DRY.

WASH LEATHER GLOVES IN THE SINK
WITH MILD SOAP AND WATER.

FOLD KNITS AND SEQUINS. DON'T HANG!

ALWAYS CONSIDER MAINTENANCE WHEN
MAKING A CLOTHING PURCHASE.

CLEAN SUITS AND OUTFITS TOGETHER
SO THAT THE COLORS CAN STAY IDENTICAL.

TURN CLOTHES INSIDE/OUT TO PREVENT
PILLING.

SWIMSUITS
Should make shoulders look wider, legs longer
Should firm, lift, or camouflage
Should never cause skin to bulge
Should allow bending, stretching, and sitting

SECRETS OF SCARVES
Use it as a head wrap
Wear it as a belt
Use it as a sarong
Wear it as a shawl
Use it as an ascot and anchor with a pin
Wear it as a fake necktie
Tie one to your purse just as the French do
Roll it as a wrist band or necklace
Dress up a hat
Wear it as a bow tie

CAN'T AFFORD A SILK SCARF?
BUY SILK FABRIC AND HEM IT.

IT TAKES ONLY MINUTES TO WORK
WITH ACCESSORY FABRICS AND WILL
SAVE $$$

SECRETS OF COLOR
BLUES MINIMIZE
REDS ENLARGE
BLACK IS MOST SLIMMING
WHITE IS FOR ACCENTING

****

ALLOW FOR A FOUR SIZE VARIANCE WHEN SHOPPING. EACH DESIGNER USES A SLIGHTLY DIFFERENT CHART.
Note: When shopping sales, be sure to look thoroughly in every size rack. Many times, the reason that the item is on sale is simply because it was size incorrectly.

****

ADD GLAMOUR WITH RHINESTONES, CRYSTALS, SILVER, AND GOLD.

****

PURCHASE FEWER THINGS BUT SPEND MORE PER ITEM.

THEME DRESSING IS ONLY ACCEPTABLE IF NOT OVERDONE.   WEAR ONE OR TWO PIECES OF ONE THEME TOGETHER. THAT'S ALL!

Example: Country/Western theme
Choose cowboy hat & jewelry or cowboy boots & shirt.

DON'T WEAR ALL THESE PIECES TOGETHER.

****

BE CAREFUL NOT TO DRESS TOO "OLD" AND DOWDY.   CONVERSELY, BE CAREFUL NOT TO DRESS INAPPROPRIATELY YOUNG. WE HAVE ALL SEEN THE OLDER WOMEN IN MICRO MINIS AND TIGHT TEE SHIRTS THAT UNFORTUNATELY EMPHASIS SAGGING BREASTS AND FLABBY ARMS.   ALWAYS KEEP AN OBJECTIVE EYE!

****

When wearing a large earring, accent it with a belt and not a necklace. It looks more well balanced.

Large beauties should coordinate an important earring with a slightly elongated pendant.

SECRETS

"I love long skirts, but they have to move! So I only purchase skirts with slits or buttons. Otherwise I can't even walk!

MARIANNE, 36/GRAPHIC ARTIST

"When I don't feel I look all that great, I throw some red on. It's the one color that picks me right up!"

CINDY, 47/TEACHER

"I keep a full length mirror by my back door. I absolutely won't go by without checking myself out. I cannot count the number of times I have been saved from going out with a ripped hem, too much jewelry, or a stain I wouldn't have ordinarily seen."

SANDRA, 30/SALES

"Before I make a major purchase in clothing, I mentally search out how I can wear it and where. If I cannot come up with at least three good answers, I put it back. It doesn't matter how much I love it or how good it looks. I know that I will regret the purchase if it lacks versatility."

TINA, 51/MEDIA BUYER

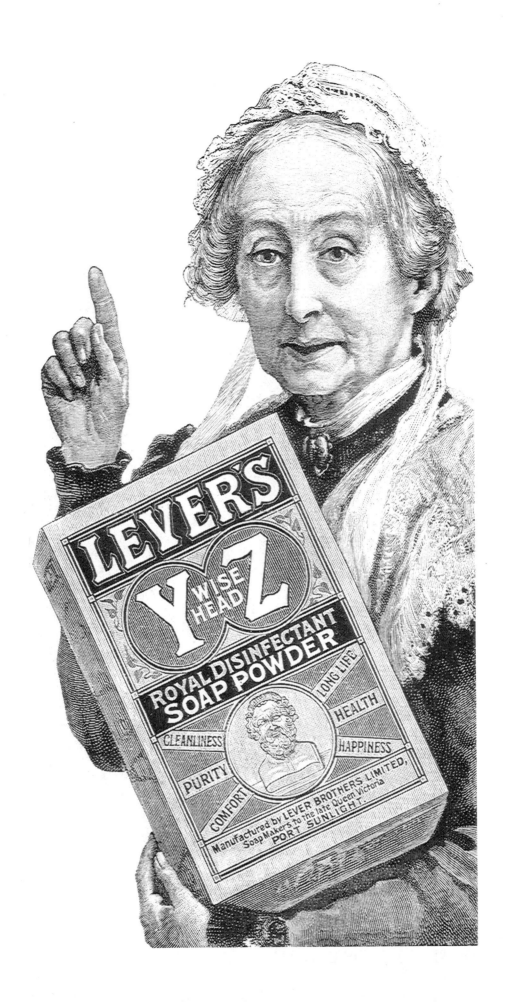

CHAPTER TWELVE

SECRETS

OF

BEAUTY

BARGAINS

Take charge of your beauty and your budget.
Start reading labels. Once you start, you will
be amazed at the savings. Many of the name brand
and cosmetic counter items contain the very same
ingredients as the drugstore/generic versions.

****

MODELS HAVE BEEN DOING IT FOR YEARS.
THEY USE LIPSTICK AS BLUSH AND EYESHADOW
AS LIP POWDER. BE VERY CAREFUL AND TEST
FOR ALLERGIC REACTIONS AND SENSITIVITY
FIRST. HOWEVER, I KNOW LOTS OF WOMEN WHO
HAVE BEEN DOING THIS FOR YEARS, AND I HAVE
TO ADMIT AFTER ALL MY SKEPTICISM,
I HAVE NOT SEEN ANY MAJOR BREAKOUTS OR
SKIN RELATED PROBLEMS.

*You can use eye pencil as a lip pencil, but
never use a lip pencil to line eyes. Lip pencils
contain ingredients that cannot be used in the
eye area. However, try creating soft blush contours
with lip pencil.*

****

The absolute best makeup organizer you can find is
an old fashioned tackle box from the hardware store.

THE REAL SECRETS OF BEAUTY

NEED AN INEXPENSIVE BURST OF YOUTH?

Purchase an old time favorite cologne.
Those sweet little scents like "Charlie" and
"Heaven Scent" are still around to take away
the years and bring back lovely memories.

****

BUTTONS CAN REFRESH, UPDATE, AND ADD ELEGANCE TO AN OLD OUTFIT.

****

Get the most out of your fragrance by applying it only
to pulse points.
WRIST, EARS, KNEES, INSIDE ELBOWS, ETC.
DON'T SPRAY THE AIR.......AIM CAREFULLY!

****

HAIRSPRAY IS A VERSATILE TOOL
Use it as a static stopper.
It also works as an emergency hose saver

PURCHASE COSMETICS DIRECT FROM
THE FACTORY AND SAVE $$$$$$$.

ORDER FROM:
COSMETIC LABORATORIES
339 48TH STREET
NEW YORK, NY.
TELEPHONE: 212-586-4144

THIS COULD BE THE VERY SAME FACTORY
THAT PACKAGES YOUR FAVORITE COSMETICS.

CREATE YOUR OWN LABEL AND STICK IT ON.
MAKE UP BEAUTY BASKETS AND USE THEM AS
PERSONALIZED GIFTS FOR FRIENDS.

THE SKIN PRODUCTS ARE FANTASTIC, AND
THE LIPSTICKS ARE THE BEST I HAVE EVER
TRIED.

PURCHASE REQUIREMENT IS $50.00 MINIMUM.
COSMETIC LABORATORIES ACCEPTS VISA
AND MASTERCARD AND GENERALLY SHIPS
WITHIN A FEW DAYS.

BEAUTY BOUTIQUE SELLS TOP NAME BRAND CLOSE OUT COSMETICS BY MAIL. SAVINGS ARE UP TO 90%.
CALL FOR A CATALOG:
800-800-0100

****

BUY PRODUCTS THAT PERFORM MORE THAN ONE FUNCTION.
One moisturizer for face and body
Witch hazel as a skin toner, cleanser, and hair degreaser
Shampoo and conditioner
Foundation and powder

****

RELY ON NATURE

Apples cut in thin slices to relieve eye puffiness
Milk or yogurt to replenish moisture
Olive oil to: remove makeup
soften rough skin
control dandruff

SOME INSURANCE COMPANIES WILL PAY FOR CERTAIN PROCEDURES:

Sunscreen if it is prescribed by a doctor

A facial if it is performed in a dermatologist's office

Some plastic surgery

****

MOST COSMETIC COUNTERS GIVE FREE SAMPLES

Many do complimentary makeovers to demonstrate products

****

GET THE MOST FROM JEWELRY

One big earring on a choker or chain is a fun and inexpensive way to use that mismate

A pair of earrings will double as a pair of cuff links

Always keep the mate of lost earrings and use them to adorn jackets, purses, and embellish plain sweaters.

SHOP HARDWARE STORES

Buy great chains for pendants and belts
Purchase organizers for cosmetics, lingerie,
belts, buttons, jewelry, etc.
Get floor wax to protect shoes and keep
them shiny

****

HAVE A CLOTHING SWAP WITH FRIENDS

You'll be surprised at how well your "biggest
shopping mistake" can look on someone else.

****

MAKE YOUR OWN STAIN REMOVER
2 Parts water
1 Part alcohol
Mix and treat garments as soon as a stain occurs.

SECRETS

" I save money by using my eyeshadow as a liner and
a contour. First, I apply my eyeshadow dry. Then
I add a little water and use it as a liner. I then change
to a thin brush and contour my eyes."

AMY, 22/MODEL

"There is no need to buy up every lipstick and eyeshadow
color on the market. I mix up my own colors according
to the current trend."

KENDRA, 31/AT HOME

"Whenever I get my hair cut, I ask my stylist to layer my
hair so that it will stay in shape longer."

VERONICA, 40/TAX SPECIALIST

"I always buy clear mascara and use it as an eyebrow groomer."

DONNA, 23/MODEL

"I shop men's departments for sweaters, shirts, and
workout clothes. It's a sad fact, but men's clothing is
priced less than the same women's items."

MARLENA, 32/RECRUITER

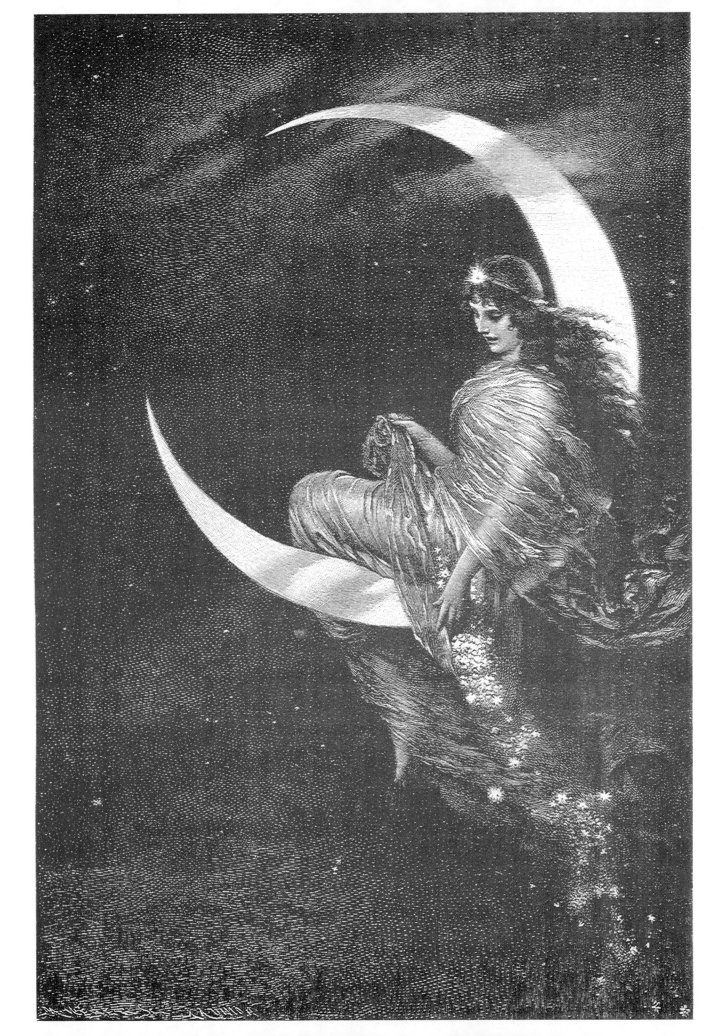

CHAPTER THIRTEEN

SECRETS

OF

TRAVEL

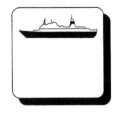

TRAVEL LIGHT!

STICK TO TWO COLORS WHEN PACKING
Add one color for dimension

EXAMPLE: BLACK AND IVORY ARE TWO COLORS THAT WORK WELL WHEN TRAVELING
Simply add a few red pieces to coordinate.

****

DRINK PLENTY OF LIQUIDS WHEN TRAVELING BY PLANE TO COUNTERACT THE DRYING EFFECTS OF "CANNED" AIR.

****

BE SURE TO TAKE ALONG PLASTIC BAGS!
USE FOR: laundry
wet suits
to prevent wrinkling between
clothing when packing

THE REAL SECRETS OF BEAUTY

ROLL, RATHER THAN FOLD WHENEVER POSSIBLE TO AVOID WRINKLING.

****

UPON ARRIVAL, HANG GARMENTS IN THE SHOWER TO STEAM.

****

ALWAYS BRING ALONG A SCARF.
> **Wear it as a sarong**
> **Hide stains**
> **Use it as a swimsuit cover**
> **Use it in place of a blouse to wear under a suit.**

****

BE SURE TO PACK:
> **Sewing kit**
> **Scissors**
> **Clothes brush**

A hairdryer can take on another life as dryer for hose, lingerie, and small stains.

SECRETS

"Whenever possible, I pack knits. They
   have never wrinkled on me, and allow for
   those extra few pounds that come with travel."
                      HANNAH, 49/COSMETICS REP

"I never wear any makeup when I travel, and I
   bring along my can of "Evian" mineral water.
   All during the trip I spritz my face to keep it
   hydrated."
                    SUSAN, 33/RECORD PRODUCER

"When I travel by plane, I phone ahead and request
   the vcgctarian meal.   It is just a little more
   bearable."
                    PAM, 45/CLAIMS ADJUSTER

"I can't stand a heavy load, so whenever possible,
   I pack sample sizes in both my cosmetics and
   toiletries."
                    KATHERINE, 60/AUTHOR

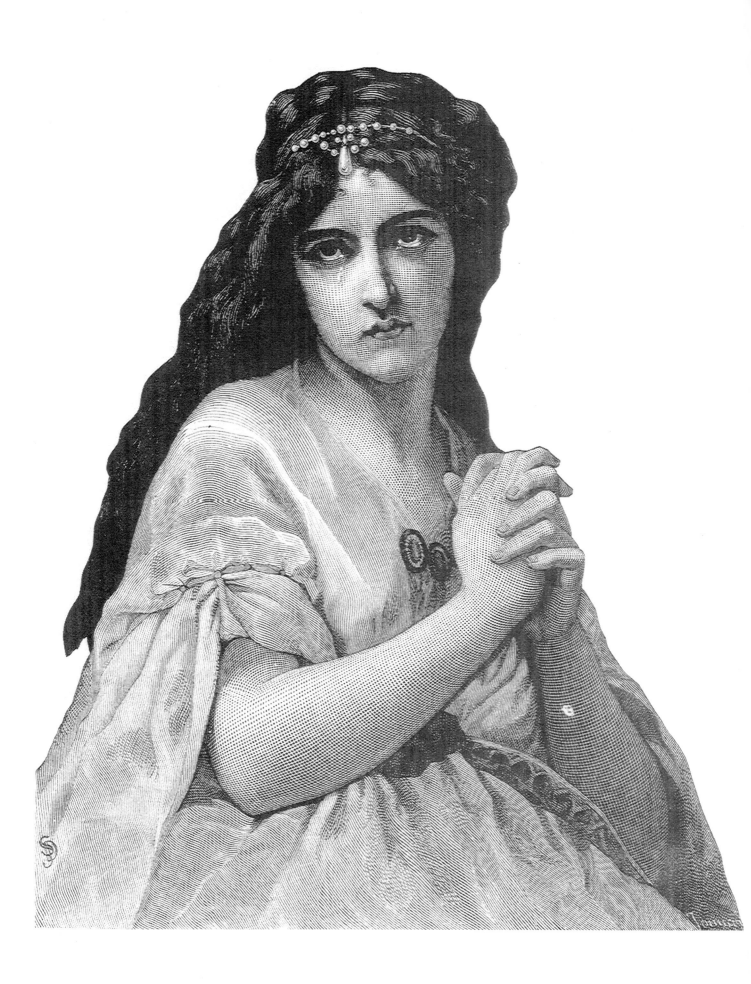

CHAPTER FOURTEEN

SECRETS

OF

BEAUTY

EMERGENCIES

THE BEAUTY CRISIS

We have all experienced it. The party that
lasted all night and it shows. The alarm didn't
ring and there's absolutely no time to get it
all together. The flu of the year is here, and
tonight's the party of the season. Here are
proven ways to look your best when
you're feeling your worst.

UNDER EYE CIRCLES

Apply concealer at least a half shade (preferably
one entire shade) lighter AFTER applying
foundation. Try a little blue eye shadow mixed
with moisturizer. Follow with foundation.

PUFFY EYES

Run a spoon under cold water and
apply to eyes briefly.

If you can plan ahead, freeze the spoons
before using.

SKIN BREAKOUT

TRUST ME ON THIS ONE!
Take any eye redness reliever and apply it
to the pimple. Take a cotton puff and saturate
it with the drops.   Press onto pimple for about
a minute.

If you are out of eye drops, take a little
toothpaste and gently dab on the blemish,
blending well.

Calamine lotion will work in the same manner.

TIRED EYES

Use navy mascara in place of black.
No navy mascara? Rub black mascara in
blue eyeshadow and apply to lashes.

Soft colors like taupe and pink are better for
fatigued eyes than stronger darker tones.

Blue liner applied inside botton lid makes the
whites of eyes appear brighter.

EXCESS MAKEUP

Sometimes makeup gets gobbed on. If you've laid a heavy hand with powder, foundation, etc. take a spritzer of water and gently spray your face. Then immediately separate a tissue and use each piece to pat your face. The residue will gently come off onto the tissue without disturbing the look. A spritz of water is also a great way to wake up a tired face.

CHAPPED LIPS

Wet lips and rub in mineral oil or petroleum jelly. Wait a couple of minutes and then blend in gloss.

TIRED FACE

Stick your face in the freezer and count to 100. Rub ice cubes over entire face, with extra emphasis on eye lid and under eye area.

HAIR PROBLEMS

Too much hairspray, gel, and mousse can easily
be diffused when there's no time to wash by wetting
down with a spritz of water and then quickly
blowing and styling dry.

For hair that's just plain dirty, dust with powder
and brush through.

RED NOSE

A little extra concealer in a darker tone
on the nose will relieve the severe redness.

Shade down the sides with darker foundation to
take away the puffiness.

CHIPPED POLISH

Dip a cotton swab with polish remover, and
pat over the chipped area to smooth it out.
Touch up with matching polish. Dry quickly
by running the nail under cold water.

BLOODSHOT EYES

Use blues to take away the redness.
Stay away from brown tones which contain
red pigment.

STAINS

White chalk covers stains on white and light colored fabric.
A black marking pen does the same for black and navy.

For an unyielding stain, cover with a decorative pin.

When there's more time, sew on appliques, or pin
with sequin decorations.

EARRINGS

If you lose a pierced earring back, pull the eraser
off a pencil and push it through the stem. It
will hold your earring in a pinch.

> PS: I find a good pencil eraser holds steadier than
> traditional earring backs with my heaviest
> earrings.

SECRETS

"When I know that I am looking tired or sallow, I
   dust a pink tinted face powder all over my face.
   It gives me a rosy glow and makes me look almost
   radiant."

                                    Jeanne, 43/Stewardess

"My eyes have a tendency to be puffy and red at the
   end of the day.   My trick is to apply cool damp tea
   bags for just ten minutes to each closed eye. The
   cheapest tea bags seem to work the best."

                                    Elaine, 26/Computer Analyst

"Sometimes I have literally minutes to go from work to
   a special event. Simply lying on my bed with my head
   hanging over the edge, gets the blood going to my brain
   and brings the color back to my cheeks."

                                    Kimberly, 32/Food Sales

"There are times when I just can't wake up. When that
   happens, I jump in the shower and take my facial exfoliator
   and exfoliate my entire body. It revs up my body, and
   I'm ready to party all night!"

                                    Lisa, 41/Retail Developer

CONCLUSION

"Beauty without grace is the hook
without the bait."
Ralph Waldo Emerson

At the risk of sounding trite, of all the women that
I have worked with, the ones who truly stood out
were the ones who didn't get carried away with
their physicality. Yes, they had that certain something,
but when I really tried to break it down, that extra
"something" was not just physical.

The point is this, no amount of makeup or clothing
will make you beautiful. The REAL secret to beauty
is to live life beautifully.   That is, to love as hard
as you can, to feel passion and compassion. And yes,
to even allow yourself to feel the pain of life.

There is a saying that "you wear your life on your
face."   Let your face show that you've lived that
life with grace and courage. Don't let beauty get
the best of you. Learn to make the most of your
looks, and then go on to all the other adventures of life.

CONCLUSION.........CONT.

Wear your beauty with dignity, style, truth, and modesty. Be happy with what you have been given and learn to appreciate not only your own loveliness but the beauty of everything and everyone you touch.

"FOR BEAUTY IS BUT THE SPIRIT BREAKING THROUGH THE SKIN."
                        Rodin/painter-sculptor

ORDER FORM

Additional copies of "The REAL Secrets of Beauty" at $17.95 & $3.00 shipping and handling.

Name:_____

Address:_____

City:_____ State:_____

Zip:_____ Phone:_____

Make checks payable to: International Image
                                   196 Main Street
                                   Wakefield, MA 01880
Charge:Visa_____ Mastercard:_____

Number:_____ Exp:_____

ORDER BY PHONE

TOLL FREE 24 HOURS A DAY!

1-800-230-9959

ABOUT THE AUTHOR

Diane Irons is a former model, Radio/TV, and newspaper journalist.   Her down to earth , consumer dedicated approach to beauty and fashion is widely known for its "down home" appeal and realistic philosophy. Her advice has been sought after internationally by media, business, and leading publications.

She is a spokesperson and consultant to TV and Radio nationally, Co-hosting lifestyle shows and personally transforming media personalities.

Diane Irons is a member of the Association of Image Consultants International, the National Speakers Association, and National Association of Radio Talk Show Hosts.